Award-winning writer, television broadcaster and author of numerous bestsellers, **Leslie Kenton** is described by the press as 'the guru of health and fitness' and 'the most original voice in health'. A shining example of energy and commitment, she is highly respected for her thorough reporting. Leslie was born in California, and is the daughter of jazz musician Stan Kenton. After leaving Stanford University she journeyed to Europe in her early twenties, settling first in Paris, then in Britain where she has since remained. She has raised four children on her own by working as a television broadcaster, novelist, writer and teacher on health and for fourteen years she was an editor at *Harpers & Queen*.

Leslie's writing on mainstream health is internationally known and has appeared in *Vogue*, the *Sunday Times*, *Cosmopolitan*, and the *Daily Mail*. She is the author of many other health books including: *The New Raw Energy* and *Raw Energy Recipes* – co-authored with her daughter Susannah – *The New Biogenic Diet*, *The New Joy of Beauty*, *The New Ageless Ageing*, *Cellulite Revolution*, *10 Day Clean-Up Plan*, *Endless Energy*, *Nature's Child*, *Lean Revolution*, *10 Day De-Stress Plan* and most recently *Passage to Power*. She turned to fiction with *Ludwig* – her first novel. Consultant to medical and cosmetic corporations in the USA and Japan and former consultant to the Open University's Centre of Continuing Education, Leslie's writing has won several awards including the PPA 'Technical Writer of the Year'. Her work was honoured by her being asked to deliver the McCarrison Lecture at the Royal Society of Medicine. In recent years she has become increasingly concerned not only with the process of enhancing individual health but also with re-establishing bonds with the earth as a part of helping to heal the planet.

Raw Energy Food Combining Diet

Leslie Kenton

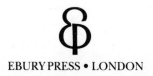

EBURY PRESS • LONDON

For Jean Morgan

who knows first hand the
blessings of food combining

1 3 5 7 9 10 8 6 4 2

Text copyright © Leslie Kenton 1996

The right of Leslie Kenton to be identified as the author of this
book has been asserted by her in accordance with the Copyright,
Designs and Patents Act, 1988.

First published in the United Kingdom in 1996 by
Ebury Press
Random House
20 Vauxhall Bridge Road
London SW1V 2SA

Random House Australia (Pty) Limited
20 Alfred Street, Milsons Point, Sydney,
New South Wales 2061, Australia

Random House New Zealand Limited
18 Poland Road, Glenfield,
Auckland 10, New Zealand

Random House South Africa (Pty) Limited
PO BOX 337, Bergvlei, South Africa

Random House Canada
1265 Aerowood Drive, Mississauga
Ontario L4W 1B9, Canada

Random House UK Limited Reg. No. 954009

A CIP catalogue record for this book is available from the British
Library

ISBN: 0 09 182001 4

Typeset by SX Composing DTP
Printed and bound in Great Britain by Mackays of Chatham plc,
Kent

Papers used by Ebury Press are natural, recyclable products made
from wood grown in sustainable forests.

Contents

Measurements & Quantities

I have given approximate measurements in the recipes as cupfuls (an ordinary cup holds about 225 ml or 8 fl oz), tablespoons, teaspoons, pinches and so on. Each time you make a recipe it will be slightly different, which is the whole fun of cooking and eating. Where measuring is important, I have given the imperial measurement as well as the metric. Most of the recipes are designed to feed four people. As the quantities are approximate, the amounts can easily be adjusted to suit your own particular needs.

In the text I have mainly used metric measurements except where the original research was done in pounds and ounces, or the statistics were quoted in gallons or feet and inches. It would be artificial in those cases to convert to metric for the sake of it. Here are a few metric/imperial equivalents which you may find useful.

Weight		Length	
28 g	= 1 oz	2.5 cm	= 1 in
125 g	= 4 oz (¼ lb)	30 cm	= 1 ft
450 g	= 1 lb	1 m/100 cm	= 39 in/3.3 ft
1 kg	= 2.2 lb	1.6 km	= 1 mile

Volume	
600 ml	= 1 pint
1 litre	= 1¾ pints
4.5 litres	= 1 gallon

Author's Note

The material in this book is intended for information purposes only. None of the suggestions or information is meant in any way to be prescriptive. Any attempt to treat a medical condition should always come under the direction of a competent physician – and neither the publisher nor I can accept responsibility for injuries or illness arising out of a failure by a reader to take medical advice. I am only a reporter. I also have a profound interest in helping myself and others to maximise our potential for positive health which includes being able to live at a high level of energy, intelligence and creativity. For all three are expressions of harmony within a living organic system.

THE PRINCIPLES

Chapter One

Simply The Best

Food combining really works. It is capable of taking excess weight off a body so simply it can be hard to believe. It can also help heal any number of long-standing ailments, from arthritis to depression, chronic fatigue, skin disorders and stomach ulcers. So good are the effects of food combining that it is little wonder the 'uninitiated' – including doctors and scientists who have never tried it – often find its beneficial results hard to swallow. How can something so simple do so much for so many? Food combining is also fun. Add the raw energy element to it and you create an unbeatable combination to help you tap into energy you never knew you had.

A little miracle of nature, the Raw Energy Food Combining Diet is the easiest and most pleasant way imaginable to shed excess fat without ever going hungry. In the process it can rejuvenate and regenerate a body and heighten vitality, making you look and feel great.

Perfect Past

Far from being some new fad, food combining diets have been tried and tested for almost two hundred years. In the last century they were used as a way of healing illness and of helping the body establish a high level of well-being. The American doctor William Howard Hay became famous for his food combining 'cures' – cures which he consistently attributed not to his own skills but to the skills of Nature herself. Once one learns to live within Her laws, he insisted, Her gifts to us are endless. Food combining was also widely taught by the Natural Hygienists in the United States and by that branch of the medical community in Europe working within the long tradition of nature-cure.

In recent times, public awareness of the importance of food combining has grown thanks to simple guide books, such as *Food Combining For Health* by Doris Grant and Jean Joice, and the American, Dr Herbert Sheldon's *Food Combining Made Easy*. Although there are often minor variations between them, each tradition which incorporates food combining as a tool for establishing radiant health or for fat loss uses the same core principles.

Aim for the Top

When it comes to weight-loss, the Raw Energy Food Combining Diet is the most effective diet of all. It adds the amazing properties of living foods to the simple technique of separating concentrated protein foods – such as eggs and cheese, meat and fish – at a meal, from concentrated carbohydrate foods – such as bread, cereals and potatoes. It is a system of living based on natural fresh foods – vegetables and fruits, wholegrains, seeds, nuts and eggs, with or without dairy products, fish, poultry and game.

Raw energy, where 50 per cent or more of your foods are eaten raw, has been used far longer than food combining – in fact for thousands of years – as a way of improving physical health and enhancing awareness throughout the civilized world. Raw Energy principles also form the basis of health and rejuvenation treatment at Europe's and America's finest health farms and spas. There, people pay a small fortune to have their bodies renewed. You can experience the same benefits of exclusive spas and health farms by using the Raw Energy Food Combining Diet at home and instead of having to pay through the nose for it, it can cost you only pennies.

Those who benefit from these spa treatments include women with cellulite, people whose metabolism has been drastically slowed down by indiscriminate use of nutritionally inadequate crash diets, and those who can't seem to shed fat at all except on starvation fare. They also include men and women who have difficulty shedding excess pounds because of food sensitivities and addictions and people who are riddled with guilt at what they see as their 'lack of self control'. By this I mean those of us who sit down to have one biscuit with a cup of tea only to find to our horror that we have devoured the whole packet. Finally, they include a few of us who, even on a healthy diet of natural foods, still have a tendency to hold on to the fat deposits in our bodies.

Go For Joy

The Raw Energy Food Combining Diet is as different from standard weight-loss regimes as a wild horse is from a taxi cab. There is nothing mechanical about it. Nor do you have to count calories or go hungry; unlike most diets, raw energy will never leave you looking haggard or feeling washed out. Instead it supports health and good looks in the highest possible way.

In fact, 'Raw energy' is an apt name for a way of eating and living which can enhance cellular vitality, restore healthy metabolism, put virtually endless energy at your disposal, and encourage your body to rebalance its biophysical and biochemical functioning so that it slowly but surely returns to its natural size and shape.

Real health cannot be measured by the absence of disease alone. It goes far beyond. Real health is not so much a *state* as a living *process* – a process through which you can make greater and greater use of your innate potential for creativity, aliveness and joy. Helping you get there is what the Raw Energy Food Combining Diet is all about.

Have you ever seen a young horse racing from one end of his field to another for the sheer pleasure of the feeling of movement in his body? Watching him move with dilated nostrils and mane blowing free can give you a real sense of what a high level of well-being – health in its broadest sense – is like: ease, freedom and above all *aliveness*.

Feel the Power

The Raw Energy Food Combining Diet can help you experience this. It has already helped thousands who have used it either because they needed to shed excess fat from their bodies or because they were less healthy than they wanted to be.

Michelangelo claimed that he never imposed any shape or form on to the piece of marble he was carving. He insisted that instead he simply used his sculptor's tools to *reveal the natural form hidden within* the stone. In many ways an overweight body is rather like his marble. Within it is hidden its vital, naturally healthy and lean form. Raw Energy Food Combining is nothing more than an efficient tool for helping to uncover it – a biological method of 'living sculpture'.

The idea that steady and permanent fat-loss can take place as a result of eating natural delicious foods while avoiding certain food combinations is going to come as a shock to some people – both nutritionists and laymen alike – who have been brought up to believe that counting calories and going hungry is the *only* way to shed excess weight. Old assumptions about weight-loss die hard. And, as you might imagine, such a diet is decidedly unpopular with the multi-million pound slimming industry, which survives on people's failures – failures which keep selling diet products almost as fast as they can be manufactured. But it can be a godsend to people who have struggled long with the battle of the bulge and who genuinely want to get rid of fat which does not rightly belong to them, and to 'run free' as the horse does.

A Whole New Ball Game

Grasp the basics of raw energy and you need never spend hours pouring over long lists of what goes with what or fretting over whether or not the salad dressing contains apple juice which may or may not go with your poached fish. The diet is easy to put into practice. It is a question of feeling your way into a new way of thinking about meals. Once you familiarize yourself with which foods belong in what general categories you will find it is child's play to plan meals.

In this little book you will find all you need – recipes, guidelines for a raw energy lifestyle, plus a fortnight of meals to inspire you. There is also a reference list of foods and categories and a chart to tell you what goes best with what. Meanwhile, here are the first principles:

- Do not eat a concentrated starch food with a concentrated protein food at the same meal.
- Try to serve only one concentrated protein food or one concentrated starch food per meal.
- Leave at least four to five hours between a starch meal and a protein one and vice-versa.

First, let's look at the rhymes and reason most weight-loss diets fail, then we'll get on to the good stuff – how to make it all work.

11

Chapter Two

The Body Strikes Back

Everybody who's ever read a diet book knows that slimming is supposed to be a piece of cake. The 'weight-loss gurus' tell us: 'One pound of fat is equal to 3,500 calories. Just tighten your belt, count your calories and subtract them from the number your body needs for energy.' (At this point they refer you to one of those dreary weight/height charts.) 'For each 3,500 calories you cut out you'll get a pound lighter. What could be easier?'

It Doesn't Work

It looks great on paper. Trouble is for most of us it just doesn't work. Why? Because nobody ever got fat just because they had a big appetite. Neither are you likely to achieve *permanent* slimness by counting calories alone.

The common myths about slimming are based on three beliefs. The first is the notion that weight-loss depends on the conscious mind balancing the body's energy intake and expenditure. The second is the idea that your body exerts no biological control over how much fat it stores. The third is the presumption that calorie-consumption is the significant factor in body-weight. All three beliefs support a multi-million pound slimming industry with all its hype, but all three are false – as dozens of scientific studies have shown.

The Slow Burn

What really determines weight-loss and maintaining it afterwards is not some abstract formula of calorie deprivation but rather how fast your body metabolizes – burns up – both the excess fat it is carrying and the food you take in day to day. This in turn largely depends upon how much cellular energy is available for the job and how efficient is your metabolism.

Sad to tell, the fatter you get, the slower your metabolic rate becomes – especially on a typical low-calorie slimming regime. In fact so inefficient can the metabolism of overweight people become that some who weigh more than 260 pounds can maintain their weight on as little as 1,000 calories a day.

The very act of going on a low-calorie diet slows your metabolism even further: your body learns to conserve energy because it feels thrown into a situation of potential starvation. This leads to rebound eating as natural hunger breaks through the constraints of personal resolve. Research carried out since the turn of the century has confirmed all of this over and over again. Yet it is something diet books still conveniently choose to ignore.

Lay the Guilt

Instead they tend to push some kind of guilt trip on people. They make you feel that you are lacking willpower or perseverance if, after ten days on some 1,000-calorie regime, you feel sluggish, slow, tired and dull, and then break your diet in a desperate attempt to restore energy and regain a sense of comfort.

Diet books are also very deceptive about the initial rapid weight-loss which most experience during the first few days on a regime. They encourage you to believe that this is good evidence that the crash diet you are on is working and that it will continue to work so long as you have the 'will-power' to keep at it. The truth is that what has been lost from your body in the first few days is not fat but water. Once this excess water from your tissues has been shed, weight-loss slows dramatically. It may even stop altogether because your metabolism has been slowed by the diet so you are simply not burning fat.

Yet it is *fat* you want to shed, not just water and certainly not lean muscle tissue. Otherwise your body will get flabbier and flabbier while your metabolism – not to mention your overall vitality – will become further depressed. There are hundreds of thousands of people who lose the same five or ten pounds over and over again only to gain it all back within a few weeks or months.

Go For Order

To shed fat *forever* you must re-establish biological and energetic *order* in your body. For it is a disturbance in this order that has caused it to accumulate in the first place. As this happens, not only does your metabolism function normally again, your digestion improves, chronic fatigue becomes a thing of the past and all those cravings that once led you to eat the wrong foods or more food than your body needs, vanish. Sounds too good to be true? Then you have not yet experienced the powers of nature-cure.

Nature-cure is an ancient system of healing which uses simple things like food and water, sleep and exercise, to establish the highest possible level of biological and energetic order in any organism. This allows an ailing or distorted body to heal itself, restoring to its owner a high level of energy, health and good looks – naturally.

The weight-loss which occurs on the Raw Energy Food Combining Diet is nothing more than simple nature-cure. It is one of the signs that your body is restoring itself to its more normal shape and function. And the power of such a diet by no means ends at paring away excess fat from an overweight body. It has also been shown to encourage the healing of any number of minor and major illnesses from rheumatoid arthritis to cancer. As any expert in natural medicine will tell you, it sets up the best possible conditions for all of this to happen. A major part of bringing all of these wonderful things about is the diet's ability to detoxify the body, while a major reason that both overweight and illness become seeded in any body is the build-up of toxicity in the system.

Toxic Traumas

The standard and widely held view of fat stored in the body is that it is fundamentally 'passive'. It just sort of sits there happily conserving energy and insulating you against cold and shock. The fact is, our fat-stores have a very *active* role to play – a protective role which it is vital to understand if you are to shed fat permanently. Fat-stores gather substances which the body experiences as toxic or poisonous and tuck them out of harm's way.

Fat cells are the perfect storehouse for these wastes since they are much less metabolically active than other cells in your body. (This is also why, once fat has been stored in cells, it can be very difficult to budge.) People who easily store fat often have difficulty dealing with these wastes. Gradually a vicious circle is created: fat-stores lower metabolic rate. Toxins continue to build up. The liver, whose job it is to cleanse them, is put

under stress. This makes it increasingly difficult to eliminate them and even more difficult for you to avoid laying down yet more fat.

Ask Any Rat

A major reason why there is so much obesity in our society is that we eat so many junk foods. Feed the same
foods to rats and 60 to 70 per cent of them get fat. It has
nothing to do with will-power, sin or guilt. Junk foods –
indeed, all refined convenience foods – are not only
nutritionally unable to support a high level of health,
they contain lots of sugar and white flour, chemical
colourings, preservatives and flavourings, all of which
encourage the build-up of wastes in the body in quantities greater than your normal waste-elimination chan-
nels can handle.

When we eat convenience foods over a period of time
two things happen. First, we end up with subclinical
nutritional deficiencies of vitamins and minerals
because so many essential nutrients have been lost in the
processing and storage of these foods. Second, wastes
accumulate in the tissues. Those of us who have inherited a genetic tendency to lay down fat-stores grow
fatter. Meanwhile, the subclinical deficiencies that we
have slowly developed in consuming typical western fare
tend to create chronic fatigue, contribute to poor skin
tone and the laying down of cellulite in women. It also
predisposes us to early ageing and further slows metabolism.

Accumulated wastes are stored mostly in the body's fat
cells. The more wastes you have the bigger your fat cells
get and the fatter you can become, whatever valiant
efforts you may make to change things. It is little wonder
that excess fat deposits have become such a problem as
we approach the millennium if you consider the toxicity

to which we are exposed. Industrial wastes fill our rivers and seas, and quite literally billions of gallons of chemicals are poured on our crops and farmlands every year. Even the fat of Arctic seals has been shown to be permeated by chemical poisons such as DDT.

Energy Equations

There is one more thing which you should know about a body which has a high level of wastes stored in its cells. Much of the available energy in such a system tends to be channelled into trying to handle these toxins instead of into keeping cells functioning at a high level of competence and efficiency as in a truly healthy lean body. In broad terms this means that you are likely to experience flagging vitality over the years and to feel that you simply can't make the effort to change things for the better.

To achieve permanent fat-loss you need rational and effective methods for eliminating toxic wastes from your body, for enhancing metabolic functions and for eliminating cravings. Once you have accomplished these goals you need to follow a way of living afterwards which will permanently help prevent their build-up. The Raw Energy Diet combines well-proven techniques of food combining with a high-raw way of eating, rich in living foods, to do all three. It boosts your metabolism and detoxifies your body while protecting your system from the build-up of acid wastes in the blood which can trigger binge eating. It alkalinizes the system and helps restore metabolic balance. It also helps resolve the energy crises which takes place when a body is overweight and digestion is overtaxed. Best of all, once the detox experience is well under way, it can bring you to experience a whole new kind of energy that will have you looking good and feeling great day after day.

Chapter Three

Energy Crisis

Your body expends more energy on the digestion of food than on any other function. This is one of the main reasons why after a big meal you can feel sluggish or sleepy and experience a lowering of vitality. What has happened is that your body has had to redirect blood (and therefore energy) away from the brain and other organs towards the gut, where your basic life-force is now busy breaking down the food you have eaten and transforming it into chemicals which can be absorbed into your bloodstream for use by your cells. In fact, the amount of energy needed to digest food is even greater than that which you use when taking strenuous exercise.

Energy Equations

For the slimmer serious about shedding fat permanently, the question of how his or her energy is directed becomes a very important issue. For an abundance of steadily available energy is needed to carry out the vital task of detoxification on which fat-loss depends. This is why all the foods you eat should be digested as efficiently as possible, both to preserve your vitality and also to make sure the quantity of toxic wastes created as by-products during the process is minimal.

The standard western meal consisting of meat-and-two-veg plus bread, potatoes and a desert represents just about the worst way you can eat if you want to lose weight. This has nothing to do with how high in calories it is either. The slimmers' low-calorie version is little better. It is the kind of meal which presents your digestive system with the most difficult of all foods for it to break down and make use of: a concentrated protein, here in the form of meat, taken together with a concentrated starch in the form of bread and potatoes.

Spanner in the Works

The human body is simply not designed to digest efficiently more than one concentrated food in the stomach at the same time. An awareness of this principle lies at the basis of virtually every tradition of natural healing.

What is meant by 'concentrated'? Any food which does *not* come into the category of a 'high-water food'. (More about the importance of the high-waters in a little while.) In other words we are talking about any food which is neither a fresh raw vegetable nor a fresh raw fruit.

Less Than Perfect

The usual response to this information goes something like this: 'How ridiculous! I have been eating meat-and-two-veg for 40 years and done perfectly well on it.' Perhaps. Yet just how well is 'perfectly well'?

If forced to be completely honest, most people who have been living in such a way for 25 to 40 years or longer will tell you they experience any number of minor digestive problems, from indigestion and flatulence to persistent hunger and being overweight, not to mention more serious rheumatoid conditions and other chronic ailments that can develop over decades of subjecting the digestive system to the heavy strain of having to cope with concentrated starches and proteins at the same meal.

The Four Horsemen

Our so-called 'normal' way of eating in the west has four basic problems when it comes to fat shedding. First, it puts great strain on your body's enzyme system – the system responsible for food breakdown and assimilation. It simply does not respect your body's enzyme limitations – and everyone's are different, depending on their genetic inheritance and on how nutritionally adequate a diet you were raised on (more about enzymes in a moment). Second, it makes heavy demands on available energy and vitality – energy which is very much needed to carry out the detoxification processes needed for permanent fat-loss. Third, it tends to produce excessive quantities of biochemical wastes which further add to the toxicity you must clear from your system if you are to be permanently free of excess fat-stores. Finally, the average diet does not supply a full complement of vitamins, minerals, trace elements, and essential fatty acids needed to support health.

So, while the human organism has a remarkable ability to adapt to difficult circumstances, and you may indeed live reasonably well on meals of concentrated starch with concentrated protein for many years, you have probably not lived this way without paying a price for it, even if the price paid so far is only decreased vitality and having to carry about with you more fat than you would like to have.

Break Down

All of the changes to foods which take place during digestion – the processes by which foods are broken down into their constituent chemical parts for use by the cells – take place thanks to enzymes. An enzyme is a kind of physiological catalyst which depends upon the presence of certain vitamins and minerals to do its job of making things happen biochemically. Each enzyme in your body is quite specific in its action. The enzymes which act upon starches do not and cannot affect either proteins or fats.

Different classes of enzymes, such as those which help break down starchy foods and those which help to break down proteins, need different chemical environments too. Starch-digesting enzymes need an alkaline environment. Protein-digesting enzymes need an acid medium: they cannot function in an alkaline environment. This is why eating high-protein foods such as eggs or meat stimulate the body's production of hydrochloric acid which, in turn, acts on the substance pepsinogen, secreted by the gastric glands, to produce the enzyme pepsin for splitting proteins. But the process only takes place efficiently in an acid environment. If there are any concentrated starches or sugars present in a meal, the accompanying alkalinity, passed on as they began to be broken down by saliva in the mouth, interferes with the process.

This can and often does result in proteins being incompletely and inefficiently digested. If the situation is severe enough it can result in 'food allergies', aches and pains and even emotional abberations – all the consequence of incompletely digested proteins (which even in minute quantities are toxic to the blood) being drawn in through the wall of the gut. On the other hand, enzymes needed to break down the starches of bread require just the opposite environment – a mildly alkaline medium. In fact they can often be destroyed even in a mildly acid milieu.

21

Starchy Truths

Starch digestion begins in the mouth, through the action of the starch-splitting enzyme ptyalin which prepares the starches for their journey into the small intestine, where their main digestion takes place. The role of ptyalin in starch digestion is extremely important: all starchy foods need to be chewed thoroughly so that saliva (which is mildly alkaline) and the ptyalin it contains can break them down sufficiently for the small intestine to carry on the good work after they are swallowed. If this doesn't happen then similar food sensitivities can occur.

The good news is that when people with food sensitivities learn the art of food combining, and practise it, many worrying and oppressive symptoms lift away. Separating concentrated protein foods and concentrated starches – that is taking them at different meals – you take the pressure off digestion, reduce the build-up of toxicity and free energy.

There is no great magic to it. By making such a change you begin to eat in a way that shows respect for the body's enzymic limitations. You are helping your body to digest your foods fully and properly – sometimes for the first time in one's life. And complete and efficient digestion is absolutely essential if you are permanently to rid yourself of the burden of unwanted fat forever. Meanwhile, plenty of fresh raw foods each day makes the job even easier.

Live for the Liver

The liver is your body's chemical factory. It carries out a myriad of essential functions, from storing vitamins and metabolizing fats to destroying unwanted materials and providing enzymes for many of your body's chemical processes. One of the most important of these functions is the breaking down or metabolism of toxic wastes. Living foods help your liver to do this job. The liver has a quite phenomenal capacity to handle detoxification. But, when it is living under constant strain as a result of having to recycle more wastes than it can manage, as well as trying to carry out all of its other functions at the same time, it can become 'overloaded' so that it simply is no longer equal to the task. Then toxins – the majority of which are fat-soluble – are simply shunted via the blood and lymph to be stored in your cells as fat.

A liver which has become chronically overloaded as its owner continues to eat the wrong kind of foods and drink the wrong kind of drinks (or to eat and drink them in the wrong combinations) will progressively send more and more toxins towards the fat cells for safe storage.

Unlike most diets, the Raw Energy Food Combining Diet works *with* the liver. That's where fruit comes in. The liver is most active between midnight and midday, so the diet uses only fruits for breakfast. Fresh fruits are so easily digested that unlike cooked foods, concentrated starches and proteins, they don't require work from the liver to handle them. This leaves your liver free to get on with the job of deep cleansing your body and shedding fat. Hence the fruit rule:

Eat fruit on its own or leave at least 20 minutes between a fruit appetizer and the next course of your meal.

Chapter Four

Life Power

Living foods have special properties for weight-loss. This is a truth which is nothing less than mind-blowing for most people. We have been brought up to consider food only in terms of chemical categories such as protein, carbohydrate, fats and fibre and to measure energy only in terms of calories.

Biochemical Blockbusters

Fresh fruits and vegetables, sprouted seeds and grains and pulses, offer the highest complement of vitamins and minerals, essential fatty acids, easily assimilated top-quality protein, fibre and wholesome carbohydrate found in nature. Such a natural complement of nutrients in superbly balanced form supplies your body with the substances it needs for its metabolic biochemical reactions to function at a high level of efficiency. This is exactly what you want to encourage – steady and permanent fat-loss.

In an overweight body, metabolism has often become sluggish and inefficient, eating the wrong foods or foods in poor combinations means vitality has been lowered and subclinical nutritional deficiencies have developed as a result of having lived on a less-than-optimal diet over a period of years.

A diet replete with living foods is the quickest and most effective way to restore balance and normality. The power that fresh, raw, living foods hold to transform life, health and good looks, lies outside the awareness of most classic nutritionists and biochemists busy quantifying the chemical characteristics of proteins, carbohydrates, and fats, with vitamins and minerals. Most of them also still tend to think in mechanistic ways.

However, the health-enhancing properties of living foods have long been tested and eulogized by highly respected European and American physicians – from Gordon Latto and Philip Kilsby in Britain, Max Bircher-Benner in Switzerland and Max Gerson in Germany, to Henry Lindlahr and J.H. Tilden in the United States.

Subtle Energies

Now, thanks to recent research into the electromagnetic and energetic properties of living plant cells, we are beginning to formulate a scientific explanation of *how* living foods can be so beneficial for enhancing health and encouraging natural weight-loss. We are beginning to understand that there is more to the metabolic improvements effected by living foods than can be measured through biochemical means alone.

All energy comes from the sun. It gets into our foods through the process of photosynthesis which plants carry out: they take in water and carbon dioxide and, thanks to enzymes they contain, in the presence of chlorophyll they produce carbohydrates (which we eat) and oxygen.

We get three types of energy from our food: kinetic energy for motion; electrical energy to maintain cell-wall integrity, muscle and nerve impulses; and chemical energy for the manufacture, storage and transport of chemicals for metabolic processes. Sunlight, through photosynthesis in plants, is the primary source of all three. This fact, although widely known and completely accepted, is too often forgotten when considering the kind of energetic information needed for high-level health which is brought to us through the foods we eat.

Sunlight Quanta

The great European physician Max Bircher-Benner, who was an expert on the healing properties of fresh live foods, always insisted that, because raw foods were still living, they contained a special health-enhancing quality of energy directly derived from the sun during photosynthesis. It is a kind of energy which is destroyed when foods are cooked or processed. When we eat these foods, he said, this special energy is passed on to us. He referred to it as 'sunlight quanta' or 'life-force'. By and large Bircher-Benner's assertions were pooh-poohed by the scientists of his day. Now physicists, many biochemists and a growing number of nutritionists, consider there is great truth in what he taught. For the biological 'information' for health and life which passes to us through the foods we eat is by no means of a *chemical* nature alone. Research into physics and the new biology demonstrates that there are other subtle forms of energy which animate organisms carried in living systems, plants and animals. These subtle energies play a central part in enhancing metabolism, rebalancing your body's functions and eliminating excess fat-stores.

Recently, thanks to the work of many highly respected biologists who have been looking both at just what kind of 'information' comes to us through the foods we eat and the subtle energies present in our environment, we have begun to measure such things as electrical fields in living cells. Evidence has emerged from this work to show that the electromagnetic or subtle energy properties of living food and of the body

26

itself are central to how well metabolism functions and how healthy we are.

In the United States, Robert O. Becker, an orthopaedic surgeon, nominated for a Nobel Prize for his work on the regeneration of tissue using electromagnetic fields, has discovered that electric conduction mechanisms in the body appear to form the basis of control systems in living organisms, and that the metabolic functions of living cells can be significantly influenced by electromagnetic means. Other scientists such as F.S.C. Northrop and Harold Saxton Burr showed the presence of what they call 'life fields' or 'L-fields' around seeds. By measuring the intensity of L-fields they are able to predict how healthy or unhealthy plants grown from them will be. They have also found that, when seeds are subjected to chemicals or heated, their fields become significantly weaker – in Bircher-Benner's terms, losses in sunlight quanta or life-force have taken place.

Living Light

Very recently, a highly respected German scientist, Fritz-Albert Popp, in collaboration with a team in China has shown – just as Bircher-Benner taught – that living cells of plants emit light in the form of biophoton radiation and that in the process of dying, as when we eat them, their cells radiate this light very intensely. Meanwhile, American cancer researcher, Herbert A. Pohl, has shown that living cells produce natural alternating-current (AC) fields which reflect biological events necessary for cell metabolism, health and growth.

Doctors and scientists working with raw energy to restore health and normal weight to patients have long been aware that many of the reasons why living foods such as fresh raw fruits and vegetables, and life-generating foods such as seeds and sprouts are so beneficial for reducing fat deposits will only begin to be explained fully when we have a better grasp of exact mechanisms by which the subtle energies in living foods act upon our bodies to encourage detoxification, to heighten enzyme activity, to improve cellular metabolism, to encourage fat-burning and to foster the quite marvellous kind of internal living sculpture which can restore some of the most neglected of overweight bodies to their natural leaner form.

It may be years before we have a full understanding of what is going on, while someone on a raw energy diet begins to reap the rewards of a slimmer, firmer body and a healthier, more energetic way of being. In fact, we will probably never have the full answer, although the work of scientists such as Becker, Popp and Pohl is rapidly taking us nearer that goal. In the meantime, however, we can make good use of the practical principles of raw energy to gain benefits. You don't need to understand everything about a motor car to make it go.

All that is important to know for now is that a raw energy way of eating encourages biochemical functions in your body to return to normal. It also fosters a high level of health and good looks. That is why, depending upon how rapidly you want to lose weight (and there are strong indications that you should not lose weight at a rate faster than two pounds a week if you intend to keep it off permanently), raw foods should form between 50 and 75 per cent of your food combining diet. Accomplishing this is easier (and more delicious) than you think.

Chapter Five

Water Margin

We are part of a living planet whose surface is over 70 per cent water. The tissues of the human body are also more than 70 per cent water. To help restore true biochemical balance and metabolic functioning to a body burdened with excess fat it is important to eat plenty of foods which are high in water content.

Living Water

Fresh uncooked fruits and vegetables and sprouted seeds, grains and legumes are high in a special kind of water – the water naturally found in living cells. The water found in living foods is invaluable in helping your body transport nutrients to all its cells and in removing toxic wastes from them. In fact, it is quite different to the water which pours from your tap. Water in living foods carries electrolytes, vitamins, organic minerals, proteins, enzymes, amino acids, carbohydrates, natural sugars, fatty acids, and other nutrients vital in the restoration of high-level functioning to the body. It helps heighten cell metabolism and makes fat burning possible.

On the Raw Energy Food Combining Diet, between 50 and 75 per cent of the foods you eat while shedding excess fat should be foods of high-water content rather than foods from which the water has been removed through drying, baking, cooking and processing.

Most of the foods we in the west eat are either not high-water foods or they have had their natural water denatured and drained away by cooking. This includes breads and pastas, meat and cheese, fried potatoes and snack foods. Even when chosen from whole natural foods and prepared without chemical additives, low-water foods should be limited while you are shedding fat. Only high-water-content foods such as fresh raw fruits and vegetables are good at waste elimination.

Limit Low-Water Foods

Low-water-content foods act differently on your body than their high-water cousins. When a food's natural water content is removed by cooking or processing, the food changes the way it acts upon the body. Low-water foods tend to clog waste elimination mechanisms and to make you feel heavy and lethargic. Low-water foods also increase cravings for more food and force you to muster the most phenomenal will-power to keep from eating too much. It is the kind of will-power that can be sustained only for limited periods, which is why so many people are off-again-on-again when it comes to weight-loss diets.

It is important to restrict the low-water-content foods you eat to no more than 20 to 25 per cent of your diet while your body is burning excess fat. Later, when you have shed your fat and your metabolism is working in top form, you can incorporate more low-water-content foods into your diet if you want to (provided, of course, you choose the most wholesome of those available).

Drink Your Fill

What about that old adage which suggests drinking

eight glasses of water a day? It is good advice for weight loss. It quite specifically helps compensate for the water-loss which occurs in the preparation of concentrated, cooked and processed foods which most people eat most of the time. But when more than 50 per cent of your foods are high-water-content and eaten in their natural fresh state, you don't need to worry so much about consuming masses of water. Of course, water acts as a natural appetite suppressant so go ahead if you fancy it. It also helps cleanse your body so drink as much fresh spring water as you like – provided, of course, you are not suffering from a kidney disease or other medical condition which precludes it.

Foods For Stamina

The rest of the Raw Energy Food Combining Diet consists of wholegrains, cooked vegetables, legumes, cooked eggs, dairy products (if you must) or fresh fish, organic meat, poultry or game. Although these foods offer little in the way of heightening cell vitality or detox-ifying the body for fat-loss, they are delicious and satisfy-ing to the palate. They are also good wholesome sources of proteins, vitamins and minerals. They are the foods which athletes or people doing hard physical work will want to eat enough of – particularly the grains. They make a rich and delicious contrast to the lighter, finer taste and feel of living foods. They will form the rest of your diet while you are slimming. Once you have lost the fat you want to shed, you can increase your intake of the stamina foods to 50 per cent or even more if you like. Many who have experimented with raw energy princi-ples, however, find that restricting the intake of heavier foods to about 30 to 40 per cent of their diet makes them feel and look better permanently.

31

Shun the Destroyers

Health-destroying foods are those which, if taken in quantity, undermine health, distort biochemical balance in the body and foster degeneration and illness. The list of foods with health-destroying tendencies is a long one and getting longer every day as scientists discover new ways in which the chemical additives in convenience and processed foods, and the hormones and drugs given to the animals from which much of our meats are taken, pose threats to human health. They include foods which have been fragmented and excessively altered from their natural state such as foods made from white flour, refined sugar, and highly processed oils and margarines – in short any food whose vital nutrients have been depleted or destroyed. Not only do you want to avoid these foods because they put a damper on the cellular life processes which are so important in heightening metabolism and burning stored fat, but also because they are the most polluting of all foods. Enough said about what to avoid. Now let's look at the upside. You will be amazed to learn what the magic living foods offer in the way of natural appetite control.

Chapter Six

Hunger Busting

Probably the worst thing any slimmer ever has to face is the feeling of never being satisfied. Persistent hunger is a major reason why people on conventional slimming diets never seem able to shed excess fat permanently. So common is it, not only with overweight people but with many of their slim brothers and sisters as well, that it is important to understand why it occurs and what can be done to get rid of it. Excessive hunger can have many causes – both emotional and physiological. But by far the most common (and the most often ignored) is chronically disturbed digestion.

Junk Food Makes You Hungry

If you have been eating irregularly, eating more than your body needs, eating foods full of chemically altered fats or which are refined and over-processed, then your natural appetite becomes distorted. To what extent depends both on the kind of digestive system you've inherited and on how badly, in physiological terms, it has been abused. Virtually every overweight body is a nutritionally starved body despite the number of calories it has consumed over the years. Its endocrine system, circulation, bones and nerves remain under constant stress. So does its digestive system.

The digestive system of a person who has been living on highly processed, chemically altered foods, or someone who chronically overeats, cannot function normally because it remains in a state of persistent stimulation. It experiences the constant overproduction of digestive juices. Good digestion is impaired. The body does not receive an adequate supply of vitamins and minerals – called *co-factors* – needed to trigger enzyme reactions. Many people in this state experience chronic hunger as a physical expression of subclinical nutritional deficiencies. The cells of their bodies are, in effect, crying out for nourishment which is not being adequately supplied. The body, in an attempt to rectify matters, seems to want to eat more and more. Another consequence is a slow-down in metabolic machinery, for every step in the body's metabolic processes depends upon good enzymic functions.

Tummy Troubles

In the beginning chronic overeating or eating the wrong kind of foods results in an over-acidic or irritated stomach. In time, however, this turns into a slack, acid-poor stomach with the kind of chronic inflammation of the intestines and bile duct that tends to accompany such a state. It is a series of events which occurs in almost every case of chronic overweight. It is also typical of people who suffer from food sensitivities.

Food sensitivities frequently accompany being over-weight. The woman who reaches for that biscuit to go with her cup of tea and finds herself eating the whole pack is experiencing the kind of allergy-addiction which forms the basis of food and chemical sensitivities. Such 'food allergies' contribute greatly to weight-gain, not only because they stimulate people to eat far too much – particularly of those foods to which they are sensitive, but also because eating foods to which you are sensitive produces a very high level of toxic wastes – far more than your liver and your lymphatic system can efficiently eliminate. So what happens? Your body lays down yet more fat-stores to lock these toxins out of harm's way.

Back to Normal

Vital factors in achieving permanent fat-loss are the restoration of your digestive processes to normal and the elimination of the kind of chronic digestive irritation which fosters persistent overeating as well as a myriad of other problems, including excessive toxicity and impaired microcirculation. The taking of oral contraceptives and a wide range of other substances, from marijuana to common prescriptive drugs, including tranquillizers, can also contribute to the toxicity, forcing fat deposits to collect on those of us with a genetic tendency towards them.

Banish the Binge

This is where binge eating comes in too – with all the guilt, disappointment and misery which accompany it. Binge eating is a typical response to the kind of biochemical anguish caused by your bloodstream having been flooded with more toxic wastes than it can deal with all at once. These same wastes in the bloodstream – most of which are acidic – are also responsible for the common dieter's nervousness, which can also trigger the eating of undesirable foods in an attempt to gain comfort or a sense of relaxation. When dieters get the typical hangovers and headaches it is simply a sign that the toxic wastes which were stored in your fat cells have now temporarily returned to the bloodstream to haunt you until they are eliminated from the body.

Bye-Bye Biscuits

Raw Energy Food Combining is the ideal antidote. First it gradually eliminates cravings by supplying your body with all the nutrients it needs (at least 50 essential nutrients are so far known. Living foods probably contain many more). Also, a diet high in raw foods calms an irritated and overactive digestive system so that its functions can gradually return to normal and you eliminate the ravenous hunger.

The result of all this is that the raw energy way of eating brings with it its own brand of natural appetite control. On a diet high in living foods the improvements which take place in digestion as well as the loss of weight itself occur steadily – quite naturally – without your having to pay attention to calories. Another wonderful thing about shedding excess fat this way is that you do not end up looking drawn or flabby. Skin and muscles become firmer and the whole body undergoes a slow process of regeneration which can seem quite miraculous to someone experiencing it.

Power For Order

Experts in the use of a high raw diet insist that the enzymes in raw fruits and vegetables also improve digestion since they *support* the body's own enzyme systems. Each food contains just the enzymes and co-factors (vitamins or minerals linked to an enzyme) needed to break down that particular food. When we destroy these enzymes by cooking or processing our foods, then our body has to make more of its own digestive enzymes in order properly to digest and assimilate them. Unless you have inherited a super-virile enzyme-replication system, without the enzymes from raw foods your body's own enzyme-producing abilities tend to wane, so that you make fewer and fewer enzymes as the years pass. Making sure your body has plenty of enzymes from raw foods is another way to help protect yourself from the food sensitivities and chronic digestive disturbances which lead to overeating.

Holistic Help

The whole issue of how digestion affects the build-up of fat-stores in the body and how it can help mobilize them is a complex one. One of the reasons why the Raw Energy Food Combining Diet is so effective is that, like any other natural form of treatment, it does not act on the body only in one or two specific ways. A diet high in living foods affects your body all over – *holistically* – in so many positive ways which interact and reinforce each other that it is impossible to delineate them all. It would even be pointless to try. The important thing is to experience for yourself just what all of these rather technical things mean in very simple terms: more energy, and freedom from constant hunger and from fatigue. It is fun to watch your body undergo its own process of living sculpture – reshaping itself from within as only a truly vital and healthy body can. Enjoy it.

Chapter Seven

A Question Of Diet

To most people, embarking on the Raw Energy Food Combining Diet is a whole new experience. They often have questions. Here are the ones most frequently asked.

Q: You say it is not necessary on the Raw Energy Food Combining Diet to eat flesh foods. But without meat, how will I be sure that I am getting enough protein?

A: It is a common misconception that if you don't eat meat, poultry, fish, seafood and game, or plenty of dairy products, such as milk, cheese and eggs, then you won't get enough protein. This is simply untrue. Meat, like eggs and cheese, is often called a 'complete' protein. What this means is that it contains all the essential amino acids – those which your body cannot make itself – in a good balance so that once its protein is broken down into its constituent amino acids it will provide your system with the raw materials needed to build its own proteins. That is, to make new enzymes and hormones and to build muscle tissue. For many years nutritionists believed that we needed to take in all of the essential amino acids at each meal in order to make proper use of them – hence the idea that a 'complete protein' was essential. Now we know that this is simply not so. You can either take in all of the essential amino acids at one meal or you can take in some essential amino acids, say, from a grain food at one meal and others from vegetables at another meal and you will still get the equivalent of a complete protein food. In other words, your body will still be able with ease to make use of the aminos these food contain to build its own proteins.

You will notice that the Raw Energy Diet is not *high* in protein but *moderate* in protein. This is for a very good reason: a prolonged intake of too much protein tends to result in deficiencies of many essential minerals such as calcium, iron, zinc and phosphorous, and even some vitamins. Also many animal studies have now shown conclusively that, while a high-protein diet brings about early rapid growth, it can also result in early and rapid ageing and degeneration. Moderate protein intake is best for long term health and resistance to early ageing.

Q: How fast will I lose weight on the Raw Energy Diet?
A: That depends on the idiosyncrasies of your metabolism and on how rapidly your body detoxifies itself. In the beginning you will probably lose weight very quickly. But this initial weight-loss will be not fat but water as your system begins to clear of toxicity. (Wastes in the tissues encourage the body to retain water in order to dilute them and render them less dangerous.) It is best to aim for no more than two pounds lost a week. This way you give your body time to change gradually: you neither risk your system being flooded with toxicity (which can make you want to eat foods in combinations you should avoid) and nor do you trigger the 'setpoint' mechanisms that spur the body to regain weight lost.

In practice you may not have much choice in the matter since many people following a raw energy lifestyle lose weight *much* faster. If you find yourself shedding weight simply increase the foods you are eating cooked – a helpful way to slow down weight loss.

Q: The diet contains a lot of raw foods and I understand that raw foods are more difficult to digest. Will they give me problems such as flatulence or loose bowels?

A: This is a common misconception. Provided they are well chewed, raw foods are *less* difficult to digest than their counterparts: this is why they form the basis of traditional dietary treatments in natural medicine. Remember, all the uncooked foods you will be eating are rich in enzymes to render them almost self-digesting. Eating them actually takes strain off your digestive enzymes. If you find you have any troubles getting used to eating more raw vegetables and fruits, chop, purée, or grate them finely using a food processor.

You may also find when you increase the level of raw foods you are eating that you are having more bowel movements than before – maybe two or three a day. This is a good sign: it means that your digestion and elimination processes are working well. Researchers find the same thing among primitive peoples living on a healthy diet of natural unrefined foods and among children raised on the same sort of diet.

Q: How expensive is a raw energy way of eating?

A: Like an ordinary diet it can be either expensive or inexpensive depending on what kind of foods you choose to buy. Obviously, if you are going to munch mangoes for breakfast and use exotic vegetables for your salads, soups and other dishes, it can be pricey. On the other hand, using the fruits and vegetables which are readily available in season, it can be very inexpensive indeed. The best of the living foods – sprouted seeds and grains – are among the most inexpensive foods you can buy anywhere, as well as being of the highest nutritional value. Living the raw energy way can be *considerably* cheaper than living on the diet of processed convenience foods which the majority of people eat these days.

Q: Do I have to eat three meals a day – even if I'm not hungry?
A: No, you don't. But you need to make sure that the foods in each of your meals are properly combined and that you have left plenty of time (four to five hours) after a protein or starch meal for it to be completely digested before you eat anything else. Many people find, after a week or two on the Raw Energy Diet that their appetite decreases dramatically. If this is the case by all means skip a meal or opt for a piece of fruit or a yogurt drink in its place.

Q: What about organic foods? Do they matter?
A: Yes, they do. Ideally most of the foods you eat on the Raw Energy Diet should be chosen from fresh, organically grown vegetables and fruits. These foods offer the highest complement of nutritional value to an organism. For most people it is just not possible to eat organic foods all the time. So eat them as often as you can.

And make at least one meal a day a living salad full of sprouts. This solves, at least in part, the dilemma about organically grown foods, for if you have grown the sprouts yourself, you *know* that they haven't been subjected to any chemical treatments. A living salad is also an excellent source of top-quality protein, essential fatty acids, and natural sugars. (When seeds are sprouted the starch in them begins to be broken down and turned into natural sugars which are easy to assimilate and provide energy to heighten your mood.) Sprouts are also brimming with life energy. It is this life energy, which is the power raw food has to transform your health, your shape, your energy and your overall good looks. As yet it is little understood by science, scientists are only beginning to measure it. Something that you will have no trouble measuring after a few weeks of Raw Energy Food Combining, however, is your firmer, slimmer shape and the new lease of life which it can bring you.

Chapter Eight

Just Do It!

That is about all there is to know. Now let's look at the 12 basic guidelines for living on the Raw Energy Food Combining Diet. Also included in this section is a quick reference chart on food combining which shows what goes best with what. Look at them often in the beginning. Soon, however, they will become second nature.

1. NEVER MIX CONCENTRATED PROTEINS WITH CONCENTRATED STARCHES

The old days of meat-and-potatoes or fish-and-chips need to be left behind. Concentrated protein foods, such as nuts, seeds, dairy products, eggs and flesh foods need an acid medium for efficient digestion; while concentrated starches, like beans and grains, potatoes, breads, cereals, yams and pumpkins need an alkaline one. When the wrong foods are mixed it delays digestion, tends to produce toxicity in the system and is responsible both for increasing appetite and digestive upsets. What you *can* get away with is the occasional garnish of protein foods or fruit foods – such as sesame seeds or raisins – in a dish to which you would never add them in greater quantity.

2. EAT FRUIT ON ITS OWN

Fruit passes through your digestive system very rapidly and needs little action by digestive enzymes in order to break it down. If you eat fruit at a meal with other foods its digestion and assimilation are slowed drastically and you can get fermentation in the gut causing indigestion, wind and discomfort. Some people even find that fruits eaten this way turn to alcohol in their stomach, affecting mind and mood. If you want to eat fruit with other food then use it as a starter and be sure to leave 20 minutes for its digestion before beginning your second course. Despite this, however, acid fruits can be used together with nuts to create a meal for lunch or supper. Both the acid or sub-acid fruits can also be eaten with cottage cheese. Sweet fruits such as bananas, raisins, dates, figs and prunes should never be put into a salad which has a concentrated protein in it. The one fruit which is rather unique in that it will combine quite well with raw vegetables in salads is apple.

3. EAT ONLY FRUIT FOR BREAKFAST

Breakfast is a fruit meal. You may eat as much as you like (provided you listen carefully to the dictates of your appetite and you masticate even the softest of fruits until the last bit of sweetness is extracted from them). Your liver – the body's most important organ for detoxification – is most active between midnight and midday. Eating fruit (which is virtually self-digesting), unlike taking in starch or protein foods, allows this detoxification process to continue unimpeded. All other foods interfere with it. You may have more fruit mid-morning if you are hungry. But make sure you leave a gap of at least 20 minutes (45 minutes for a banana) before you begin your midday meal. You must leave 4–5 hours after a main starch or protein meal before eating fruit again and do not drink fruit juice between meals (except as a starter, leaving plenty of time before the rest of your meal, or as a mid-morning snack if you wish).

4. MUNCH A SALAD ONCE A DAY

A living salad based on home-grown or store-bought

sprouted seeds and grains is the mainstay of the Raw Energy Food Combining Diet. While it is by no means absolutely essential that you base one of your meals each day on a salad, this is the best possible way to get optimal support for rebuilding cells and tissues, rebalancing bio-chemical processes, and restoring normal metabolism. Sometimes, of course, this is not possible – for example, when you are having to eat in restaurants all the time – but then you can replace the living salad with a big dish of lightly cooked fresh vegetables, served with a side-dish of grains, a soup or a protein food or simply with a couple of slices of wholegrain bread. But the more often you are able to make a living salad the focus of the meal, the sooner you will reap the rewards of your new lifestyle.

5. CHOOSE THE BEST

This doesn't mean spending lots of money: it means being fussy when you go to the greengrocer and always choosing foods which are fresh, as much as possible whole (such as wholegrains), and eaten as close as possible to their natural state.

6. SHUN OVERPROCESSED AND UNCLEAN FOODS

Chemically fertilised foods or foods which have been excessively processed to alter their natural state are depleted of nutrients. They often contain additives such as artificial colourings and flavourings which are potentially harmful. These include foods such as white breads, sugar, most meats, sweets, coffee and all the ready-in-a-minute convenience foods that fill the shelves of our supermarkets. These are the most polluting of all foods.

7. MAKE STAPLES YOUR SIDE-DISHES

These are the stamina foods. They include wholegrains and cooked vegetables, legumes and dairy products, fresh fish, organic meat, poultry and game. Both delicious and satisfying, such foods are good sources of sustained caloric energy (particularly the grains) and useful as a provider of proteins for the body's amino-acid pool. They also make a beautiful contrast to the lighter, finer taste and feel of living foods. Use them with pleasure but in moderation. The best way to do this is to serve them as side-dishes at your high-raw meals. This is a brand new and very healthy twist to the traditional practice of making meat and cooked vegetables the focus of a meal which is then eaten with a side-salad. These cooked foods become the side-dishes to the living main recipes.

8. SWIM WITH THE WATER MARGIN

Your body is 70 per cent water. For it to detoxify itself and to encourage the restoration of normal functioning on a cellular level as well as in the system as a whole, 50 to 75 per cent of what you eat each day needs to be chosen from the high-water foods: fresh fruits, sprouts, and vegetables eaten raw. This is probably the easiest guideline of all to keep to, for when you are having only fruit for breakfast and making one meal a day a living salad or supersalad it just about takes care of itself. But there may be days when you find you have eaten more of the staple foods than you should because of being invited out or having to eat in restaurants. Then it can be helpful to make the next day an all-raw day where you have fruit for breakfast as usual, a living salad for lunch, and then another fruit dish or a supersalad for dinner.

9. DON'T EAT BETWEEN MEALS

(Except, that is, between breakfast and lunch – fruit – if you are really hungry). Your digestive system must have time to complete the digestion of a meal before you put anything else into it. Four or five hours need to elapse between lunch and dinner. Otherwise digestion is not complete and increased toxicity can ensue. Do drink as much spring water or herb teas between meals as you like. And if a meal is delayed beyond four or five hours after

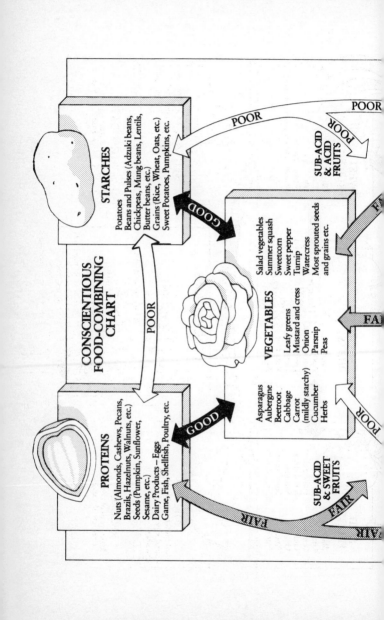

CONSCIENTIOUS FOOD-COMBINING CHART

STARCHES

Potatoes
Beans and Pulses (Adzuki beans, Chickpeas, Mung beans, Lentils, Butter beans, etc.)
Grains (Rice, Wheat, Oats, etc.)
Sweet Potatoes, Pumpkins, etc.

VEGETABLES

Salad vegetables
Summer squash
Sweetcorn
Sweet pepper
Turnip
Watercress
Most sprouted seeds and grains etc.

Leafy greens
Mustard and cress
Onion
Parsnip
Peas

Asparagus
Aubergine
Beetroot
Cabbage
Carrot (mildly starchy)
Cucumber
Herbs

PROTEINS

Nuts (Almonds, Cashews, Pecans, Brazils, Hazelnuts, Walnuts, etc.)
Seeds (Pumpkin, Sunflower, Sesame, etc.)
Dairy Products – Eggs
Game, Fish, Shellfish, Poultry, etc.

SUB-ACID & ACID FRUITS

SUB-ACID & SWEET FRUITS

POOR

POOR

POOR

GOOD

POOR

GOOD

GOOD

FAIR

FAIR

POOR

FAIR

FAIR

FAIR

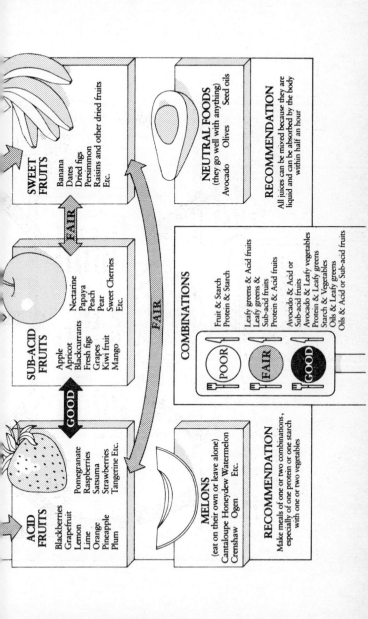

ACID FRUITS
(eat on their own or leave alone)

Blackberries
Grapefruit
Lemon
Lime
Orange
Pineapple
Plum

Pomegranate
Raspberries
Satsuma
Strawberries
Tangerine Etc.

GOOD ↔

SUB-ACID FRUITS

Apple
Apricot
Blackcurrants
Fresh figs
Grapes
Kiwi fruit
Mango

Nectarine
Papaya
Peach
Pear
Sweet Cherries
Etc.

FAIR ↔

SWEET FRUITS

Banana
Dates
Dried figs
Persimmon
Raisins and other dried fruits
Etc.

FAIR

NEUTRAL FOODS
(they go well with anything)
Avocado   Olives   Seed oils

RECOMMENDATION

All juices can be mixed because they are liquid and can be absorbed by the body within half an hour

COMBINATIONS

POOR
Fruit & Starch
Protein & Starch

FAIR
Leafy greens & Acid fruits
Leafy greens &
Sub-acid fruits
Protein & Acid fruits

GOOD
Avocado & Acid or
Sub-acid fruits
Avocado & Leafy vegetables
Protein & Leafy greens
Starch & Vegetables
Oils & Leafy greens
Oils & Acid or Sub-acid fruits

MELONS
(eat on their own or leave alone)
Cantaloupe Honeydew Watermelon
Crenshaw Ogen Etc.

RECOMMENDATION

Make meals of one or two combinations, especially of one protein or one starch with one or two vegetables your last meal you can have a piece of fruit or two to tide you over. Otherwise stick carefully to your meal times.

10. CHOOSE YOUR CONDIMENTS

Read labels on what you buy and make sure that any commercial salad dressings, condiments and seasonings contain no chemical additives, sugar or preservatives. They will only increase the toxicity in your body. Use raw honey for sweetening and then only occasionally and in small quantities.

11. BE CREATIVE

Don't forget, the suggested menus which follow are merely guidelines. Play about with them and make them your own. Figure out ways of getting your favourite foods into your meals. You might be surprised to find just how many of the recipes in the section which follows will appeal to others in your family as well. If you make a living salad for yourself make a little side-salad just like it to go with the chop you may be cooking for your husband. Many a family member has been gently drawn into a healthier way of eating and living by taste alone. Never preach. Have fun with it. If you do it may well eventually turn out to be fun for the rest of your family as well.

12. MAKE TIME FOR EXERCISE

Be good to yourself and make sure that, no matter what kind of mountains you have to move to do it, you set aside a space in your life of at least 30 minutes in a day, four times a week, for exercise – brisk walking is best – and relaxation. This is an absolute must since it spurs the release of toxicity, firms the body and improves your ability to handle stress. In due course it will become a joy as well. But a little effort is required *now* to make it possible.

Take a close look at the Raw Energy Food Combining chart. Use it like a map to steer you through the new territory of your lean and energetic lifestyle.

THE PRACTICE

Chapter Nine

Go Easy

So you've met the principles of Raw Energy Food Combining, it's now that all the fun begins. For, unlike the usual low-calorie regime with its minute portions of processed foods, the Raw Energy Food Combining diet offers you as much as you want to eat from nature's cornucopia of delights. The beauty and the texture of fresh foods prepared in simple yet attractive ways is, for me, one of the great pleasures of life. When I first began exploring Raw Energy Food Combining for myself, I was amazed to discover three things. Firstly, these foods which were so good for me were also more delicious than any I had eaten before. Secondly, they were simple to prepare. Finally, this way of eating offered such an extraordinary variety of taste, aroma, colour and texture that I was never bored.

All Change

Raw Energy Food Combining is far more than just a programme for weight-loss: it is a lifestyle for high-level well-being – a way of living that will help prevent premature ageing, illness and fatigue. And it is not something which you follow for a period of weeks until you have shed your excess fat, then return to the same old eating habits which caused you the fat problem in the first place. Think of the Raw Energy experience which you will be having in the next few weeks as a transition between the way you *were* living and a better, more energetic and satisfying lifestyle of the future – a lifestyle which will protect you permanently from ever having to deal with a fat problem again. During the next few weeks you will be going through a kind of metamorphosis which will help balance your body's biochemical functioning and put you in harmony with your natural body-cycles. Once this metamorphosis has started, the process of detoxification will continue uninterrupted. And, so long as you continue to make the Raw Energy Food Combining principles the guidelines by which you live, fat-loss will take place automatically – as a natural consequence of the whole process – until your body happily readjusts itself to its most comfortable and natural weight. One of the great blessings of this metamorphosis is that, the further along you are in the change process, the more energy and initiative you will find you have to continue. It is rather like getting yourself into the opposite of a vicious circle: each positive thing that you do reinforces yet further positive change.

One Man's Meat

Here you will find recipes for soups, salads, dips and dressings, vegetable dishes and all the other basic dishes which fit easily into the raw energy way of living. You will not, however, find recipes for fish, poultry, game, seafood and eggs – for two reasons. First, most people already know how to prepare these foods. Second, although they are foods which you should by all means eat and enjoy if you want to, they are in no way *essential* to the transformation which will be taking place within the next few weeks. Indeed, eating too many flesh foods or eating them too often may interfere with the detoxification process. However, if you enjoy them by all means eat them – but make sure that they are prepared simply, without the addition of starch-based sauces, and make sure you eat only one flesh food at a meal. The best way to prepare flesh foods is, as I say, simply – by grilling, baking or poaching. Free-range eggs can be made into delicious omelets or hard-boiled and then grated and sprinkled on your salads.

You can create your own delicious dishes by combining eggs or flesh foods with light crisp salads and serving them hot or cold. But probably you won't want to eat flesh foods more than three or four times a week. They are very concentrated proteins and also low-water foods. Don't forget that for effective detoxification and efficient fat-loss you need to make sure that 70 per cent of what you eat comes from the high-water foods such as fresh raw fruits and vegetables and sprouts.

The Raw Energy Kitchen

Most of the things you need in order to prepare delicious recipes for your new raw energy lifestyle are things which you probably already have in your kitchen. The one machine I consider essential is a food processor. You can get by without a blender as the food processor can do many of the same things but, if you happen to have one, it too can be useful. When buying either it is most important that you buy good strong machines which will stand up to heavy demands.

A good food processor is a real blessing to a raw energy lifestyle. These machines have many varied and remarkable attachments including, usually, a blade, several graters of different sizes, slicers and shredders. The blade attachment is great for grinding nuts, seeds and wheat and other sprouts, homogenizing vegetables for soups and loaves, and making dressings and dips. In fact, many of these can also be done in the blender, but if they are gooey they tend to get stuck around the blade and you can spend five minutes trying to scrape out your dessert with very little to show for it. The blade of the food processor, by contrast, is removable and easy to scrape, so you lose very little.

The other food-processor attachments are terrific for making salads. You can prepare a splendid raw energy salad in about five minutes with the help of these friends. Experiment with grating, finely slicing and shredding all kinds of vegetables because, believe it or not, vegetables actually taste different depending on how they are cut up!

Keep It Simple

The following are helpful if you don't have a food processor and a lot of other electrical equipment like blenders or juice extractors. However, you may find that using these hand-powered alternatives you are a little limited in the variety of recipes you are able to prepare.

- Food processors: there are several hand-operated types which perform either chopping functions or grating/slicing, etc.; some are rather cheaply made, so keep an eye out for a sturdy one.
- Hand meat/grain grinder or coffee grinder: for mincing grains and grinding seeds and nuts.
- Pestle and mortar: for grinding herbs, spices, etc.
- Hand grater: the box kind with several different facets is best.
- Citrus reamer: the well known 'lemon squeezer'.
- Salad basket: the kind made of wire which you go outside and swing around your head.

In a raw energy lifestyle, the things that matter most are, of course, the foods themselves. And there are so many different ways of preparing them that you can probably turn the lack of a food processor or other equipment to your advantage if you let it push you towards discovering even more creative ways of serving the splendid natural foods which you will be eating.

This little book contains scores of recipes for you to sample. I hope that they will serve as inspiration to you to create your own; if you do I would love to hear about them. The recipes are simple and portions in them are loosely defined: most will serve about four people. I encourage you to cut them in half, alter them in any way you fancy to include your own favourite ingredients, and even enlarge them if you wish when you feel particularly hungry and want to eat more. But remember that you must always chew your foods *completely* so that you get every morsel of pleasure you can out of them. Remember, too, that you must stop eating immediately when your appetite signals to you that you've had enough. DO NOT OVEREAT.

Look on the next few weeks as a period of transition, take a deep breath and make the leap into Raw Energy.

Here we go.

Chapter Ten

Shop Hound

Now it is time, with Raw Energy principles in mind, to think about stocking your larder. Many of the foods you will be using on the Raw Energy Food Combining Diet you probably already have. Others can be found in supermarkets, healthfood stores and wholefood emporiums. And, of course, most of the fresh foods are readily available at your supermarket or local greengrocer. The sprouts you will use for your living salads can be bought in some supermarkets and in healthfood stores. But they are so much more delicious if you grow them yourself (see pages 66-71).

The list of fresh wholesome food is very large indeed. It contains over 150 quite common foods and, of course, there are the herbs, the wild salad foods, and the more exotic fruits and nuts which you can get if you want to take the trouble to look for them.

Let's take a closer look at some of the different types of food that are available and the specific foods which you may want to choose from to create a raw energy food combining way of eating for lasting fat-loss.

Fruit Magic

The 'great eliminators', fresh fruits are high in vitamins, minerals and enzymes, all of which help detoxify your system at a rapid rate. The gentle acidity of most fruits can dissolve waste substances in the tissues and help carry them away. Fruit also helps stimulate metabolism. Make at least one meal a day an entirely fruit meal. And for maximum weight-loss it is a good idea to spend at least one day a week detoxifying your body on a single fruit. Probably the best fruit (in a temperate climate like Britain) is the apple. Fruits to choose from include:

apple	mango
apricot	mulberries
banana	nectarine
berries	ogen melon
blackberries	orange
blackcurrants	pawpaw (papaya)
blueberries	peach
cantaloupe melon	pear
cherries	Persian melon
cranberries	persimmon
Crenshaw melon	pineapple
fresh figs	plum
gooseberries	pomegranate
grapefruit	prunes
grapes	raspberries
honeydew melon	redcurrants
kiwi fruit	satsuma
kumquat	strawberries
lemon	tamarind
lime	tangerine
lychees	watermelon

The Yummy Demis

Avocados, tomatoes, peppers and cucumber are actually classified botanically as fruits. However, they are most frequently used as vegetables. In fact, they do combine well with other fruits. You can put avocado together with mango, for instance, or cucumber together with oranges very successfully. These vegetable fruits also combine well with neutral vegetables and with the starchy carbohydrates such as rice, other grains, and potatoes.

The vegetable fruits are best eaten raw. Except for the avocado they tend, like most fruits, to pass through the stomach very quickly. The vegetable fruits are:

avocado	peppers (red, green yellow)
cucumber	tomatoes

Go Live

These foods contain important organic minerals and vitamins. They too help eliminate stored toxicity in the system. Each day you can eat as much raw salad as you like. You can use these foods to supply the necessary minerals such as calcium and iron as well.

Generally speaking, most vegetables mix well, both with concentrated proteins and with concentrated starches. Those which are stored (rather than eaten fresh), however, are very high in starch and should be used only for starch meals. Recommended fresh raw vegetables include:

alfalfa sprouts	cos lettuce
artichokes	dandelion leaves
asparagus	dill
bean sprouts	endive
beans – fresh	fenugreek sprouts
beetroot	garlic
beet greens	greem beams
Brussels sprouts	green peas
cabbage	Jerusalem artichoke
carrots	kale
cauliflower	kohlrabi
celery	lamb's lettuce
Chinese leaves	leek
chives	lettuce (all kinds)
collards	marrow
corn-on-the-cob	mung bean sprouts

mustard greens
mushrooms
onion
okra
parsnip
parsley
pumpkin
potatoes
radish sprouts
radishes
salsify

scallions (shallots)
spinach
spring onions
sweet potato
Swiss chard
turnip
turnip greens
watercress
yam
yellow beans

Gifts From the Sea

If you have never used the sea vegetables for cooking, this is an ideal time to begin. Not only are they delicious – imparting a wonderful, spicy flavour to soups and salads – they are also the richest source of organic mineral salts in nature, particularly of iodine. Iodine is the mineral which is necessary in order for the thyroid gland to work efficiently. As your thyroid gland is largely responsible for the body's metabolic rate, iodine is very important for fat-loss.

I like to use powdered kelp as a seasoning. You will find it in some of the recipes. In fact, I use it in many more – to add both flavour and minerals to salad dressings, salads, soups and so forth. I am also very fond of nori seaweed, which comes in long thin sheets. It is a delicious snack food which you can eat along with a salad or at the beginning of the meal: it has a beautiful, crisp flavour. I like to toast it very, very quickly by putting it under a grill for no more than 10 or 15 seconds. It is also delicious raw.

Get to know some of the sea vegetables and begin to make use of them. Your nails and hair will be strengthened by the full range of minerals and trace elements such as selenium, calcium, iodine, boron, potassium, magnesium, iron and others, which are not always found in great quantities in our ordinary garden vegetables. So will the rest of your body.

You can use nori seaweed to wrap around everything from a sprout salad to cooked grains in order to make little pieces of vegetarian *sushi*. It's often a good idea to soak some of the other sea vegetables such as dulse, arrame and hiziki for a few minutes in enough tepid water to cover. This softens them so that they can be easily chopped to be put into salads or added to soups. Sea vegetables are available in healthfood stores and in oriental food shops. Recommended ones are:

arrame	kelp	nori
dulse	kombu	wakami
hiziki	laver bread	

About to Sprout

The sprouted seeds, grains and legumes are truly life-generating and are the very basis of the diet. These foods contain life- and health-enhancing energies which appear to potentialize and mobilize dormant life forces in the animal organism eating them. At least one meal a day should consist of a large dish of raw foods. This can be a large soup or a salad containing the sprouted seeds and the grains or both. See the sprouting chart on page 76. Recommended ones include:

adzuki (aduki)	curly cress	sesame
alfalfa	lentil	sunflower seeds
buckwheat	mung	triticale
chickpea	mustard seeds	watercress
cress	radish	wheat

Go Nutty

These living foods are very concentrated sources of body-building protein and are also rich in natural oils.

They should be eaten regularly as part of the diet but never in great quantities. They are more difficult to digest than fresh fruits and vegetables and are often best used chopped very finely and sprinkled on to salads. When you're eating nuts or seeds at any meal it is often best not to eat other concentrated foods at the same meal. Try these:

almonds	hazelnuts	pumpkin seeds
brazils	marrow seeds	sesame seedss
caraway seeds	pecans	sunflower seeds
cashews	pine kernels	walnuts
coconuts	poppy seeds	

You will notice that peanuts (groundnuts) are not listed here. This is because they are in fact legumes and not nuts at all. They are an excellent source of vitamin B3 and biotin but are also very acid-forming. They should be treated as a concentrated protein and eaten only in small quantities, always raw, never roasted and never heavily salted.

Staffs of Life

Grains were the first food which man cultivated, and they have formed a major staple ever since. They are not strongly eliminative but they are well-balanced foods which contain the nutrients needed for good health – particularly the B-complex vitamins. Wholegrains are also an excellent source of fibre and of sustainable energy. They are important foods for athletes and for very active people.

On the Raw Energy Food Combining Diet you can include your 'quota' of grains by preparing side-dishes such as millet, brown rice, buckwheat (a seed rather than a grain but often classified together with the grains) or wholemeal pasta to go with your vegetables and salads. Or you can eat a slice or two of any good wholegrain bread with your neutral or starch meal. Most slimmers find that they are better off eating rye or pumpernickel breads – the European darker, heavier, natural breads – than the usual wholewheat. This is because wheat contains a high percentage of gluten which in many people tends to clog the intestines. Despite its quite high bran content, wholemeal bread can cause intestinal discomfort which can lead to excess appetite and also, surprisingly, to constipation in some people. There are also some excellent grain breads and crackers on the market which you can buy.

The grains themselves make wonderful additions to starch soups or may be cooked on their own as a side-dish.

Recommended breads and biscuits include:

wholegrain pitta bread	rye crisp
pumpernickel bread	100 per cent rye
home-made bran muffins	Scottish oatcakes
wholecorn tortillas	wholegrain chapatis
wholegrain bagels	

Recommended grains and grain products include:

barley	kasha
bulgar wheat	millet
corn meal	pasta (wholegrain)
couscous	rice (brown)

Take Your Pulse

The legumes/pulses are unusual foods in nature in that many of them are both concentrated starches and proteins. As such (with the exception of lentils) they can be quite difficult for many slimmers to digest. Therefore on the Raw Energy Food Combining Diet few legumes are used – except, of course, in sprouted form. The one which is commonly used unsprouted is the lentil – red, brown, green or black.

Legumes often contain a trypsin inhibitor, a substance which blocks the action of some of the enzymes which break down protein in your body. Because of this, legumes should never be eaten raw, because then a proportion of the valuable amino acids they contain cannot be used. Trypsin inhibitors are destroyed when the legumes are cooked, and sprouting neutralizes the trypsin inhibitors as well. (The sprouting of lentils and other legumes and grains also destroys other harmful substances such as phytic acid [see page 68.])

Tofu – soybean curd – is a very high-protein food which is low in fat and much favoured in the Orient. It can make an interesting addition to a salad dressing or as the basis of a protein salad.

The Dodgy Dairies

Ideally any dairy products that you eat on the diet should be unpasteurized and low in fat. This is becoming extremely difficult in Britain. However, there are some excellent unpasteurized goats' milks available from which you can make goats' yogurt, and there are some very good simple white cheeses such as ricotta and low-fat cottage cheese; although these are pasteurized they are low in fat and can be used as an adjunct to a living salad or as part of another dish. It's best to stay away from the heavy, hard cheeses: not only are they fairly acidic, they are also very rich in fat.

Free-range eggs, particularly if they are fertilized, are themselves living foods (especially when raw) and certainly have a part to play in the Raw Energy Food Combining Diet. However, they offer the highest utilization of protein of any food. You need to eat very few eggs to benefit from them.

Yogurt can be an extremely good food on the diet too – particularly if it is home-made (see pages 72-5 for instructions.) Sheep's yogurt is my favourite. Natural yogurt helps restore the healthy intestinal flora which have been damaged by eating a diet too high in refined foods or by taking antibiotics or other medication.

Dairy products of note are:

butter (small amounts and best salt-free)	feta cheese
	free-range eggs
cottage cheese and other low-fat natural white cheeses such as Petite Suisse	(preferably fertilized)
	goats' yogurt
	natural/unsweetened yogurt
cows' yogurt	sheep's yoghurt

Greet Meat

There is no necessity to eat flesh foods at all on the Raw Energy Food Combining Diet: you will get a full complement of proteins from the mixes of your sprouted seeds and grains, nuts, the occasional egg and low-fat cheese. However, if you do choose to eat flesh foods then they should be those foods which have had the least processing. This excludes most meats, such as beef, lamb and pork, since the flesh of these animals is very high in fat and also tends to contain a high level of chemical contaminants which you want to avoid. So, if you choose to eat flesh foods, opt for free-range poultry, organic meats, game and seafood, all of which are lower in saturated fats and less likely to be contaminated.

One animal-food recipe worth remembering is a Free-Range Omelet stuffed with whatever sprouts you have available; dress with Light Vinaigrette, sprinkle the top with tamari, and serve.

Meat and fish vary tremendously in quality depending upon their freshness and on how much exposure the creatures have had to chemicals, growth hormones, artificial feeds and so forth. You can choose from:

Cornish hens	game
free-range chicken	organic beef, lamb
fish	or pork
free-range turkey	seafood

Sparkle & Spice

Seasonings such as sea-salt, vegetable bouillon powder, tamari, herbs, spices and mustard have an important role to play in the Raw Energy Food Combining Diet. They bring great variety of taste to different sauces, soups, vegetable dishes and salads. Choose the very best and use them in creative ways.

Sauces and Condiments

Honey
Raw honey is honey that has not been heated or thinned. It is rich in certain vitamins, minerals and enzymes, but is a very concentrated food and should therefore be used only in very small quantities.

Miso
A fermented soya-bean paste which is rich in digestive enzymes and high in protein. It can be used for seasoning soups and sauces. It is also a delicious addition to dips for crudites and salad dressings.

Mustard
Either Dijon or Meaux.

Sea-salt
The only type of salt which you should use – and use it *sparingly*.

Tamari
A kind of naturally fermented soy sauce made by fermenting soya beans, wheat and sea-salt. It is a good seasoning for soups, salads and dressings.

Tahini
A paste made from ground sesame seeds which is delicious and very nutritious. It is a protein condiment.

Vegetable Bouillon Powder
An excellent natural seasoning made from vegetables, sea vegetables and sea-salt. It can be used in salad dressings, soups, vegetable dishes – I use it in very many of my recipes instead of salt. It is available from healthfood stores or direct from Marigold Health Foods Ltd, Unit 10, St Pancras Commercial Centre, 63 Pratt Street, London NW1 0BY.

Spices and Herbs

I grow many herbs in my own garden and use them constantly in my sauces, my soups and my salads. However, I also use packaged seasoning, particularly when the fresh herbs and spices are not available. Here are some herbs and spices that I strongly recommend for use in the Raw Energy Food Combining Diet:

allspice	lovage
anise	mace
basil	marjoram
bay leaves	mint
cardamom	mustardseed
caraway seeds	nutmeg
cayenne	oregano
celery seeds	paprika
chervil	parsley
cinnamon	pepper (black)
cloves	rosemary
coriander	sage
cumin seeds	summer savory
curry powder	tarragon
dill	thyme
fennel	turmeric
ginger (preferably fresh)	winter savory

Thirst Quenchers

Juices

If you are lucky enough to have your own centrifugal juice extractor (see page 150) you can make some excellent drinks from vegetables and fruits – for instance, by mixing raw carrot juice and raw apple juice half and half. Building upon this formula you can add a little cucumber or mustard and cress or celery or fresh tomatoes to create some delicious cocktails.

Because these juices contain no fibre the vegetables and fruits mix very well with each other, and they will be absorbed within 15 to 20 minutes of drinking them. They make an excellent beginning to a meal.

If you are not fortunate enough to have a juice extractor you can buy some very good European vegetable and fruit juices which have been processed at low heat. 'Biotta' make several good kinds. In Britain 'Aspell' apple juice is a very good low-heat-processed natural apple juice.

Water

Drink only water that has been filtered, in order to remove some of the chlorine and heavy metals it contains, or bottled spring water.

Tea and coffee

These do not belong on the diet because both of them can leave large quantities of toxic residues in the system. Instead, try Café Hag (decaffeinated), some of the excellent coffee substitutes such as Lane's Dandelion Coffee, or Pioneer, or some of the excellent herb teas. I particularly like those made by 'Celestial Seasoning': my favourites are their Cinnamon and Rose, Sleepytime, Red Zinger and Almond Sunset. You can add a teaspoonful of raw honey for sweetening if you want to.

Chapter Eleven

Sprout It

To me, nothing surpasses the best of home-made food. And there are two kinds of foods in the Raw Energy Food Combining Diet which are particularly good when you do it all yourself: sprouts and yogurt. They are also so simple to make that it seems a shame to buy them. We'll look at each in turn.

Despite all our scientific knowledge, nobody can yet explain exactly how one tiny seed is able to grow into a plant: this is part of the mystery and the power of nature. But the process is something you want to make good use of if you are to rid yourself permanently of unwanted fat. Living foods are unique in nature simply because they have the potential to create new life when germinated.

A major reason why sprouted foods are so helpful for slimming is that they help break through that vicious circle of inertia, which fat people tend to experience, and to replace it with a sense of vitality and energy which makes a lot of hitherto impossible things possible – like feeling positive about yourself or having enough energy to go out for long walks or jogs each day – and enjoy them. Sprouted biogenic foods are able to supply enzymes, minerals and vitamins as well as subtle life energies which encourage metabolic efficiency and provide your body's metabolic pathways with the raw materials needed to function in top form. Just how is by no means completely understood. But what is known about the mysteries and magic of sprouts is enough to leave your head spinning at these little miracles of nature.

Secrets of Sprouting

The most important staple of the raw energy salad, sprouts, are easy to grow any time and just about anywhere. All you need to start your own indoor germinating 'factory' are a few old jars, some pure water, fresh seeds/grains/pulses, and an area of your kitchen or a windowsill which is not absolutely freezing. Sprouts form the basis of living salads, soups and dressings. Most sprouts are neutral foods and can combine with either proteins or starches.

Home-made sprouters
There are two main ways to sprout seeds – in jars and in seed trays. Let's look at the traditional way first, then at the way I find easiest and best.

A simple and cheap sprouter can be anything from a bucket to a polythene bag. The traditional sprouter is a wide-mouthed glass jar. Some people like to make it all neat by covering the jar with a cheesecloth or a nylon or wire mesh and securing it with a rubber band, or using a mason jar with a screw-on rim to keep the cheesecloth in place. But I find the easiest and least fussy way is simply to use open jars and to cover a row of them with a tea-towel to prevent dust and insects from getting in.

Start here
- Put the seed/grain/pulse of your choice, for example, mung, in a large sieve. (For amount to use see the chart on page 76 and remember that

most sprouts give a volume about eight times that of the dry seeds/grains/pulses.) Remove any small stones, broken seeds or loose husks and rinse your sprouts well.

- Put the seeds in a jar and cover with a few inches of pure water. Rinsing can be done in tap water, but the initial soak, where the seeds absorb a lot of water to set their enzymes in action, is best done in spring, filtered or boiled and then cooled water, as the chlorine in tap water can inhibit germination and is also not very good for you.

- Leave your sprouts to soak overnight, or as long as is needed.

- Pour off the soak-water – if none remains then you still have thirsty beans on your hands, so give them more water to absorb. The soak-water is good for watering houseplants. Some people like to use it in soups or drink it straight, but I find it extremely bitter. Also, the soak-water from some beans and grains contains phytates – nature's insecticides, which protect the vulnerable seeds in the soil from invasion by micro-organisms. These phytates interfere with certain biological functions in man including the absorption of many minerals (including zinc, magnesium and calcium), and are therefore best avoided. The soak-water from wheat, however, known as 'rejuvelac', makes a wonderful liquid for preparing fermented cheese and is very good for you.

- Rinse the seeds either by pouring water through the cheesecloth top, swilling it around and pouring it off several times, or by tipping the seeds of the open-topped jars into a large sieve and rinsing them well under the tap before replacing them in the jar. Be sure that they are well drained either way as too much water may cause them to rot. The cheesecloth-covered jars can be left tilted in a dish drainer to allow all the water to run out. Repeat this morning and night for most sprouts. During a very hot spell they may need a midday rinse too.

- Return sprouter to a reasonably warm place. This can be under the sink, in an airing cupboard or just in a corner not too far from a radiator. Sprouts grow fastest and best without light and in a temperature of about 21°C (70°F).

- After about three to five days, your sprouts will be ready for a dose of chlorophyll if you want to give them one. Alfalfa thrive on a little sunlight after they've grown for two or three days but mung beans, fenugreek and lentils are best off without it. Place them in the sunshine – a sunny windowsill is ideal – and watch them develop little green leaves. Be sure that they are kept moist and that they don't get too hot and roast!

- After a few hours in the sun most sprouts are ready to be eaten. Optimum vitamin content occurs 50–96 hours after germination begins. They should be rinsed and eaten straight away or stored in the refrigerator in an airtight container or sealed polythene bag. Some people dislike the taste of seed hulls such as those that come with mung sprouts. To remove them simply place the sprouts in a bowl and cover with water. Stir the sprouts gently. The seed hulls will float to the top and can be skimmed off with your hand.

Make it big

Now for my favourite and simplified method using seed trays. I find that, with the great demand of my family for living foods, the jar method simply doesn't produce enough. Also, for sprouted seeds, you have to rinse twice a day while tray sprouts need only a splash of water each day. This is a very simple way to grow even very large quantities easily.

Take a few small seed trays (the kind gardeners use to grow seedlings, with fine holes in the bottom for drainage). When germinating very tiny seeds, such as alfalfa, you will need to line your seed tray with damp, plain white kitchen towels. For larger seeds the trays themselves are enough. Place the trays in a larger tray to catch the water that drains from them. Soak the seeds/grains/pulses overnight as in the jar method, then rinse them well and spread them a few layers deep in each of the trays. Spray the seeds with water (by putting them under the tap or by using a spray bottle) and leave in a warm place. Check the seeds each day and spray them again if they seem dry. If the seeds get too wet they will rot, so be careful not to overwater them. Larger seeds such as chickpeas, lentils and mung beans need to be gently turned over with your hand once a day to ensure that the seeds underneath are not suffocated. Alfalfa seeds can be simply sprinkled on damp paper towels and left alone; after four or five days they will have grown into a thick green carpet. Don't forget to put the sprouts in some sunlight for a day or so to develop lots of chlorophyll. When the seeds are ready, harvest them, rinse them well in a sieve and put them in an airtight container or sealed polythene bag until you want them. To make the next batch, rinse the trays well and begin again.

Tips and tricks

Some sprouts are more difficult to grow than others, but usually if seeds fail to germinate at all it is because they are too old and no longer viable. It is always worth buying top-quality seeds because, after removing dead and broken seeds, and taking germinating failures into account, they work out better value than cheaper ones.

Also try to avoid seeds treated with insecticide/fungi-cide mixtures such as those which are sold in gardening shops and some nurseries. Healthfood shops and whole-food emporiums are usually your best bet. At wholefood emporiums you can buy seeds very cheaply for sprouting in bulk. It is fun to experiment with growing all kinds of sprouts from radish seeds to soya beans, but avoid plants whose greens are known to be poisonous such as the deadly nightshade family, potato and tomato seeds. Also avoid kidney beans as they are poisonous raw.

Some of the easiest to begin with are alfalfa seeds, adzuki (aduki) beans, mung beans, lentils, fenugreek seeds, radish seeds, chickpeas and wheat. Others include sunflower seeds, pumpkin seeds, sesame seeds, buckwheat, flax, mint, red clover and triticale. These lat-ter can sometimes be difficult to find or to sprout – the 'seeds' must be in their hulls and the nuts must be really fresh and undamaged. Good luck!

Yogurt is a Snap

As a health-giving protein food, yogurt is most impor-tant for its action on the intestinal flora. The lactic-acid bacteria it contains synthesize B vitamins, which are needed in the intestines. The acid medium they create in the colon is unfavourable for the growth of patho-genic and putrefactive bacteria. In fact, laboratory studies show that many pathogens, such as those caus-ing typhoid fever, dysentery and diphtheria lose their virulence when placed in yogurt and are killed even in yogurt whey. This is one of the reasons why yogurt is very good for curing gastro-intestinal disorders. It is also useful in restoring the digestive tract after the use of antibiotics, which destroy all the intestinal bacteria (including the friendly ones) plus many of the B vita-mins.

Yogurt is far more easily digested than milk. One reason is that the milk protein in it has been partially broken down by the bacteria. Perhaps even more important is the breakdown of lactose (milk sugar) to lactic acid which occurs when milk is made into yogurt. This is of significance because many people (whether they know it or not) have difficulty digesting milk. In adulthood they lose the ability to produce the enzyme lactase so that they can no longer break down lactose; this results in lactose intolerance. Undigested lactose remains in the intestines and attracts water. It can cause bloating and excessive flatulence as well as abdominal pains and diarrhoea. But many people who experience difficulties with drinking milk can eat yogurt without any problem. Another advantage to yogurt is that the calcium and phosphorus contained in it are much more available for absorption than in milk.

The best yogurt is made from sheep's or goats' milk. Cows' milk is harder to digest and more mucus-forming. Goats' and sheep's milk and yogurt can be bought at healthfood shops while plain natural cows'-milk yogurt can be found in supermarkets.

Make it Scrumptious

Yogurt-making is really a lot easier than most people think. You don't need fancy yogurt-makers, thermometers, sterilizing fluids, etc. All you need is some milk, a container, a warm place and a 'starter'.

It is really worthwhile to try making your own yogurt because, provided you can get good fresh goats' or sheep's milk to make it from – or even powdered skimmed cows' milk – it needn't be heated above body-temperature, and so you retain the health-giving enzymes in the milk. Also, home-made yogurt is so much tastier than bought. One reason is that manufactured yogurt is not as fresh as it could be. It also sometimes contains stabilizers and preservatives which prevent it from spoiling too quickly. The result is a slightly tangy sour taste which can put people off yogurt. The natural home-made kind is actually sweet-tasting. With a little practice you can very quickly become an expert at making it.

Milk

Goats' and sheep's milk are best. You can buy a large quantity frozen and keep it in your freezer if you have the space. Soya milk can also be used. If you want to make cows'-milk yogurt you can use low-fat skimmed milk powder. This is slightly better than whole milk and is very simple to use as it does not need to be boiled.

Container

Use whatever you happen to have as a container. Either an earthenware pot, crock or casserole, heat-resistant wide-mouthed glass jar, wide- mouthed thermos flask or a stainless-steel cooking pot will do. But it should be made of an inert material: no aluminium or flaky lacquered dishes. The container should have a lid.

A warm place

There are many ways of getting round this one. Country stoves such as Agas are ideal. The container can be stood directly on an upside-down saucer or a wire cooling tray on top if the stove is too hot. An airing cupboard or an oven heated to 120°F (50°C) and then switched off are both good. If you choose a radiator, or the warm area at the top back of the fridge, the container should be wrapped in a blanket or towel for insulation. You can also use a polystyrene bucket or picnic hamper with a lid to make an 'incubator', or even make a simple 'hay box' using a couple of cardboard boxes: one is used as a lid to fit over the other with the yogurt container in the centre surrounded by blanket/hay/newspaper or any insulating material. The ideal temperature to be maintained is 90–105°F (32–40°C). You can also use a wide-mouthed thermos which will retain the blood heat you need to culture the yogurt for six to eight hours and is ideal.

Starter

There are two kinds of starter – plain yogurt or powdered culture (the latter can be found in some health-food shops). The yogurt starter can be of any sort of milk (cows'-milk if you can't get hold of goats' or sheep's). It should be plain, natural yogurt with nothing added. Read labels! Some things advertised as yogurt in supermarkets in fact contain no lacto-bacteria at all. And don't buy fruit yogurt: it doesn't work and it also contains sugar. Once you make your first batch of yogurt you can use your own yogurt as a starter indefinitely. In fact, the yogurt gets tastier each time you do. If it starts to become sour then use a fresh starter.

Two Pints of Yogurt

- Heat two pints (1 litre) of milk to just below boiling point (small bubbles should just be appearing at the edges of the pan). You can buy a round china disc that goes in the bottom of the pan and begins to rattle at the point when you need to remove the milk from the heat. (If you're using fresh goats' or sheep's milk from a good supplier, you can skip this step and just warm the milk to body temperature.) You can also use 'soya milk' to make yogurt. In this case you need only heat to blood heat before adding the culture.

- Leave the milk to cool to the temperature where you can comfortably put a finger into it and keep it there. It should feel neither hot nor cold – about blood-heat.
- Rinse your container with boiling water. This sterilizes it, which is important because you don't want any foreign bacteria in your yogurt. It also warms it and helps keep the milk at a constant temperature while the yogurt is incubating.
- Pour the milk into the container and add your culture. You will need a generous tablespoonful of yogurt for each pint of milk or 'soya milk' you use. If you are using milk powder, mix it with pure blood-heat water in a blender – the more powder you use, the thicker your yogurt will be – then add your starter.
- Stir the culture in well. This is important to distribute the bacteria – otherwise you can end up with a lump of yogurt swimming in a dish of milk. (Be sure that whatever you use to stir the mixture has been rinsed in hot water too.)
- Place the lid on the container, or cover with cling film (the yogurt bacteria are anaerobic). Put the container into your warm place and leave for about six to eight hours. The faster the yogurt curdles, the sweeter it will be. If it hasn't cultured in this time (it can take up to 10 hours), leave it longer.

Goats'- and sheep's-milk yogurts tend to be thinner than cows'-milk ones. If you get a rather watery yogurt first time, don't worry: it is still delicious and it tends to get thicker each time a new batch is cultured. Experiment with the temperature of your warm place. Yogurt keeps in the refrigerator for up to about a week. Use it with fruit to make delicious yogurt drinks, or for soups and salad dressings.

SPROUT IT

Variety	Soak Time	Dry Measure	Days to Harvest	Sprouting Tip
Alfalfa	Overnight	3 tbsp	4–5	Grow on wet paper towel – place in light for last 24 hours
Chickpea	Up to 24 hours	2 cup	3–4	Needs long soak; renew water twice during soak
Fenugreek	Overnight	½ cup	3–5	Pungent flavour
Lentil	Overnight	1 cup	3–5	Earthy flavour
Mung	Overnight	¾ cup	3–5	Grow in the dark – place in light for last 24 hours

Chapter Twelve

Breakthrough

Here is a fortnight of menus to get you started. You will find the recipes in the chapters that follow (use the index) – except in the case of the flesh foods. I have given alternatives three or four days a week depending upon whether or not you want to eat the flesh foods. If you do, remember that the best ones are game, fish, seafood organic meats and free-range poultry. If you don't, then simply take the other option. Lunch and supper are interchangeable.

These menus are only guidelines to get you started. Play with them and create your own raw energy foodstyle around what you like best – the best menus are your own!

DAY ONE

Breakfast

Fresh fruit, either *au naturel* or made into a fruit frappé or fruit salad. Have as much as you like but chew it well so that you extract all the goodness and flavour from each bite. If you are hungry you may have another couple of pieces of fruit or a fruit drink mid-morning as well. Should you choose melon as your fruit, don't mix it with other fruits – eat it on its own.

Lunch
Sprouted Lentil Salad
and
Barley Mushroom Soup

Dinner
Green Glory Salad
Baked Leeks and Pecans
or
Grilled Chicken Breast with Lemon
Baked Parsnips

DAY TWO

Breakfast
Same as on day one

Lunch
Red Witch Salad
Yummy Brown Rice

Dinner
Live Avocado and Tomato Soup
Mange-tout and Almond Stir-Fry
Mixed Green Side Salad with French Spice Dressing

DAY THREE

Breakfast
Same as on day one

Lunch
Fresh Orange Juice
(leave 20 minutes before main course)
Bulgar Salad with Endive

Dinner
Gazpacho
Easy Vegetable Curry

or
Curry made with Organic Lamb
Small Sprout Salad with Italian Dressing

DAY FOUR

Breakfast
Same as on day one

Lunch
Green Light Salad
Racy Red Cheese
Avocado Delight Dressing

Dinner
Spicy Shish-Kebab
Kasha *or* Brown Rice
Sliced Tomatoes with Sprout Splendour Dressing

DAY FIVE

Breakfast
Same as on day one

Lunch
Baked Potato Stuffed with Blue Dolphin Salad
Horsey Tomato Dressing
or
Snappy Apple Salad with Cottage Cheese

Dinner
Ruccola Salad
Light Vinaigrette Dressing
Aubergine Paté
or
Poached Salmon with Fresh Parsley and Lemon Juice
Baked Onion

DAY SIX

Breakfast
Same as on day one

Lunch
Celebration Salad
or
Pineapple Treasures Served with Nuts

Dinner
Living Soup
Vegi-Stroganoff

DAY SEVEN

Breakfast
Same as on day one

Lunch
Spring Gardens Salad
Nut Mayonnaise *or* Pink Yogurt Dressing
or
Berry Muesli

Dinner
Tomato Treasures
Split Pea Soup
or
Braised Vegetables

DAY EIGHT

Breakfast
Same as on day one

Lunch
Greek Delight Plus Salad
or
Summer Red and White Fruit Salad

Dinner
Root-Is-Best Salad
Celery Special Dressing
Free Range Omelet
or
Organic Steak

DAY NINE

Breakfast
Same as on day one

Lunch
Large bowl of crudités served with
Soya Cottage Cheese, Tahini Mayonnaise
or
Raw Houmus

Dinner
Watercress Salad
Italian Dressing
Crunchy Stir-Fry
Millet

DAY TEN

Breakfast
Same as on day one

Lunch
Corn Soup
Cress Special
Horsey Tomato Dressing

Dinner
Charismatic California Salad
(with a sweet Cashew Cream to which you
have added a tablespoonful of raw honey)
or
Ratatouille and Raita Salad

DAY ELEVEN

Breakfast
Same as on day one

Lunch
Courgette Tomato Soup
Branton's Booster
Light Vinaigrette *or* Italian Dressing
or
Organic Lamb Chops
Green Salad with Italian Dressing

Dinner
Small Cress Special Salad
Barley Pilaff
Minty Peas

DAY TWELVE

Breakfast
Same as on day one

Lunch
Crudités served with
Potato Supreme Salad

Dinner
Sliced Cucumbers
Light Vinaigrette
Sesame Stir-Fry
Kasha

DAY THIRTEEN

Breakfast
Same as on day one

Lunch
Greek Delight Plus
or
Stir-Fried Vegetables with Organic Beef

Dinner
Slice of Melon (don't forget the 20 minutes!)
Easy Vegetable Curry
Yummy Brown Rice *or* Millet

DAY FOURTEEN

Breakfast
Same as on day one

Lunch
Scottish Pine Salad

Dinner
Red Witch Salad
Curried Pumpkin Soup
or
Braised Vegetables
or
Prawns grilled in a little oil and garlic

Now that we've looked at some sample menus, let's explore the recipes themselves.

Chapter Thirteen

Breakfast To Go

Breakfast is sheer bliss; the easiest part of Raw Energy Food Combining. It consists of nothing but fruit. The reason for this is simple: the digestion of fruit is so easy that it demands only a tiny fraction of the energy needed to break down other foods in your body. All fruits – except bananas, dates and dried fruit, which stay in your stomach for about 45 minutes or so – are in your stomach no more than 20 to 30 minutes. There they are broken down so that vitamins and minerals are almost instantly made available for absorption into the bloodstream. And, because they require so little energy for digestion, the energy available to your body is not disturbed when you eat them, so it can continue to focus on the elimination processes which are central to the detoxification of your system and encourage fat-loss.

Fruit Stands Alone

Fruit does not stay in the stomach for very long, it is best eaten on its own. It should certainly not be eaten together with other foods, such as protein foods or most starchy foods – although nuts and low-fat dairy products such as yogurt and cottage cheese can combine quite well with some fruits. (See the chart on pages 46-7) Neither should you eat fruits immediately after a concentrated protein or starch food. However, when you eat them on an empty stomach – the best way for fruits to be eaten –their effect is extremely positive.

Fruit has the highest water content of any food: between 75 per cent and 90 per cent of all fruit consists of natural mineral water. Raw fruit also contains a beneficent mix of ions (electromagnetically charged particles). This can help enhance metabolic functions on a cellular level and cleanse even long-standing residues from your tissues and encourage weight-loss.

These are some of the reasons to begin each day with fruit. This can either be fruit in its simple original form – an apple or two, fresh berries, apricots or melon – or it can entail using fruits to create delicious and even elaborate fruit dishes to delight your aesthetic senses. The practical advantages of eating fruits on their own are obvious. Breakfast takes almost no time at all and certainly no preparation if it consists of something as simple as a handful of apricots or a couple of figs, an apple or two or half a grapefruit. For most people this will suffice. But when you begin to explore the different delicious possibilities of dishes that can be made from fruit they can seem too tempting to resist preparing them – especially for beautiful Sunday breakfasts in bed!

Detox Dramas

It is not only because they require little digestion, so that the energy otherwise used to digest food can be used to continue the detoxification process, and because they help heighten the micro-electrical potentials of cell tissues that fruits are so efficient for cleansing the body. They are also good detoxifiers because they contain a high percentage of carbon. The high carbon content of fruits encourages them to act as incinerators of waste matter in the digestive system as well as in the bloodstream, the internal organs, the skin and, on a cellular level, elsewhere throughout your body.

Fresh fruits are also alkalinizing to the system – even the 'acid' fruits. This is very important for your body since it can encourage cellular repair and help counteract the acidic wastes eliminated from the cells which tend to build up when you are under stress (most of the byproducts of stress are acidic). Not just raw fruits but also raw and cooked vegetables, help increase your resistance to stress and fatigue thanks to their ability to render the blood slightly more alkaline.

A few people claim that fresh fruit is difficult for them to digest. This should not be the case provided you never eat it *with* any other kind of food or *following* anything else. Occasionally someone will experience a sense of bloating and wind if they are not used to eating fresh fruits when, at first, they begin eating them for breakfast. This is because the fruits' powerful cleansing ability encourages rapid elimination of toxicity, and in the process can temporarily create wind and bloating (it can also be because of a severe *Candida albicans* infection). But this is not a common experience. When it does occur it usually clears up within a day or two. If it does not you should consult a qualified nutritionist or a doctor trained in nutrition.

Eat Your Fill

Every morning choose whatever fruit appeals to you and eat as much of it as you feel comfortable with. You need not worry about the calories that your fruit contains. Simply listen to your own 'inner voice' to tell you when you've had enough and stop there. And remember to chew each bite of the fruit you eat thoroughly. This complete chewing is the only way you will derive the full benefit from whatever you're eating.

Above all *don't let yourself overeat* . . . but don't let yourself undereat either. Eat enough fruit that you feel satisfied. Be pleased with what you're eating, enjoy it, and remember that the fruits you're eating are playing an important part in the detoxification process that will allow you to lose excess fat permanently. If in the middle of the morning you find that you feel hungry again, by all means have another piece of fruit – or even two. Remember, though, to leave at least 30 minutes after eating a piece of fruit before you begin your lunch.

The lists of fruits you can choose from is a long one – just look at the list on page 55. The dried fruits, such as figs, peaches, coconut, pears, pineapple, prunes, apricots, raisins, sultanas and apples are too concentrated for slimmers (remember the 70 per cent rule): they are best left alone until you have achieved the desired fat-loss: then you can incorporate them into your diet.

Occasionally you can turn your fruits into fresh fruit juices, although it is far better to take the fruit as a whole since the natural fibre in fruit also plays an important part in the detoxification process. A delightful way of getting the best of both worlds is to mix a particular fruit, say a mango, in a blender together with a little orange or apple juice. It makes an absolutely delicious fresh fruit frappé which you can either drink or make thick enough to eat with a spoon. Such a drink is a meal in itself – as are many of the fruit dishes you'll find on pages 90-7. They make delightful total-meal recipes which are particularly good for light suppers. Use them often. Meanwhile, here are the important points about fruit breakfasts.

The Breakfast Guide

- Eat as much fruit as you like up to one pound at a time, but make sure that you chew it very thoroughly.
- If you are hungry in the middle of the morning have another piece or two of fruit.
- Steer clear of the dried fruits until you have eliminated all the excess fat you want to shed.
- Eat bananas only if they are very ripe and you are very hungry and feel that you want a heavier food, and remember that they take longer to digest: allow 45 minutes after eating a banana before eating your lunch.
- *Never overeat* . . . but likewise never undereat. Eat just as much as you need to feel satisfied.

Chapter Fourteen

Get Fruity

Among the greatest pleasures of Raw Energy Food Combining are some of the beautiful fruit dishes you can prepare as total meals. An all-fruit meal is a wonderful way to end the day – an ideal light supper. Also, a fruit salad with a little fresh yogurt makes an energizing lunch, and I love making a quick fruit frappé instead of a meal in the middle of Summer when everyone longs for something cool and frothy. Here you will find some of my family's favourite fruit treats. Some are suitable for breakfast since they are made of fruit only; others are designed as lunch or dinner dishes.

These are only my personal inventions. Fruits offer such a wide range of colours, textures and flavours, and there are so many ways of using them, that you will no doubt create even more beautiful dishes on your own. When you do I would love to hear about them!

Remember that you can always start your lunch or dinner with a simple all-fruit appetizer such as a piece of cold melon or a bunch of sweet grapes, or a glass of freshly pressed fruit and vegetable juice. But, if you do, allow 20 to 30 minutes before beginning your next course.

In all the recipes used in this book, C = cupful; tbsp = tablespoonful; tsp = teaspoonful

Tropical Delight

I have an absolute passion for tropical fruit – I think I could live on it! This is a particularly tasty combination of some of my favourites.

1 papaw, peeled, seeded and sliced
2 ripe bananas, sliced lengthways twice then chopped into small pieces

1 mango, peeled and diced
¼ C apple juice
30 ml (2 tbsp) coconut flakes
dash of nutmeg

Put the fruits into a bowl. Add the apple juice (you may use concentrated apple juice with a little spring water added if you prefer) by pouring over the fruit. Serve immediately garnished with coconut flakes and sprinkled with nutmeg.

Tropical Promise

A simple yet delicious dish which I enjoy when papaws are readily available.

2 bananas
2 small papaws, peeled and seeded
45 ml (3 tbsp) desiccated coconut flakes

30 ml (2 tbsp) raisins which have been soaked in water for a few hours

Slice bananas and papaws and arrange on a salad plate. Sprinkle with coconut flakes and raisins. Serve immediately.

Summer Red-and-White Fruit Salad

A stunningly beautiful fruit salad which makes a luscious full-fruit meal.

1 C cherries, pitted and halved
1 C plums, pitted and quartered
1 C raspberries
outer leaves of a lettuce
375 g (12 oz) low-fat cottage cheese

½ pineapple (outer skin cut off, flesh cut into rings, core removed)
15 ml (1 tbsp) finely chopped pineapple mint or apple mint

Combine the cherries, plums and raspberries and mix well. Arrange a few lettuce leaves on a plate and lay pineapple rings on top. Place a scoop of cottage cheese in the centre of the ring and pour the other fruit mixture over the top and sprinkle with fresh mint.

Spiked Apricot Supreme

Another delicious fruit meal – not a breakfast dish – is this delightful and spicy combination of apricots, coconut and cinnamon.

6-8 ripe apricots, pitted and cut into small pieces	For the Sauce
	3/4 C dried coconut
1 ml (¼ tsp) cinnamon	*a little spring water*
1 ml (¼ tsp) allspice	*5 ml (1 tsp) honey*
15 ml (1 tbsp) raw honey	*5 ml (1 tsp) fresh vanilla essence*

Blend half of the chopped apricots in a blender to which you add the cinnamon, allspice and honey. Arrange the rest of the apricots in glass dishes and pour the apricot spice mixture over them. To make coconut cream, mix the dried coconut (make sure you do not buy the kind that has sugar added to it) with enough spring water in a blender to get the consistency of heavy cream. Add the honey and vanilla essence and continue to mix. Spoon the coconut cream on to the apricot dish and serve immediately.

Poire Suprême

Who would ever have thought such a splendid dish could be concocted from the simple pear?

4 pears, cored and sliced thinly but not peeled	*juice of 2 lemons*
	3 drops of oil of peppermint
30 ml (2 tbsp) raw honey	*½ C blackcurrants*

Place the thinly sliced pears in a dish. Combine the honey, lemon juice and oil of peppermint in a glass and mix well with a spoon. Pour over the pears. Chill in a refrigerator for 30 minutes, then garnish with blackcurrants and serve immediately.

Charismatic California Salad

A sunshine spectacular of the acid fruits, with avocado used as a source of protein and essential fatty acids. You can make this salad in any size – small if you want a small snack meal or very large indeed to create a large and extremely filling fruit meal.

1 orange
1 satsuma or tangerine
1 pink grapefruit
1 ripe avocado

3 or 4 large leaves from the outside of a lettuce
15 ml (1 tbsp) lemon juice
a few strawberries (optional)

Peel, remove the seeds and section the citrus fruits and cut the segments into bite-size pieces. Peel and chop the avocado and strawberries (if desired) and mix together with the other fruits. Add lemon juice and toss gently. Line a bowl with lettuce leaves and place mixed salad in the centre. Serve immediately.

Snappy Apple Salad

This is a simple and pleasant fruit salad based upon apples and grapes. It can be served as a main meal either with nuts, such as pecans, almonds or hazels and a scoop of low-fat cottage cheese or a dish of fresh yogurt. I particularly like it with sheep's yogurt as a light supper.

3 sweet apples, chopped
1 orange, peeled, sectioned and cut into bite-size pieces
1 satsuma or tangerine, peeled, sectioned and cut into bite-size pieces

1 C fresh green grapes
2.5 ml (½ tsp) allspice
pinch of cinnamon
125 g (4 oz) nuts or low-fat cottage cheese or yogurt

Combine all the fruits and spices. Mix and allow to chill in a refrigerator for 15–30 minutes. Serve the fruit in a large flat dish and top with yogurt, low-fat cottage cheese or chopped nuts. Serve immediately.

Pineapple Treasures

The perfect dish for a splendid Sunday brunch. Pineapple treasures not only look wonderful, their flavourful combination of succulent berries and fresh pineapple almost melts in your mouth.

1 ripe pineapple
1 ripe avocado
1 C fresh raspberries or
   strawberries or blackberries
   or 1/3 C of each
a little honey (optional)

30 ml (2 tbsp) chopped fresh
   pineapple mint or
   spearmint
30–45 ml (2–3 tbsp) chopped
   almonds or hazelnuts or
   cashews (optional)

Cut the pineapple in two lengthwise, scoop out the insides, cutting the pineapple flesh into cubes. Toss it together with the other fresh fruits, including the avocado; you may add a little honey if you wish. Refill the pineapple shells with this fruit salad mixture and garnish with the mint. May be served for breakfast or as a main meal. As a main meal you can sprinkle with two to three tbsp of chopped almonds, hazelnuts or cashews.

Stuffed Avocado

Another unusual and delightful main meal. Avocados combine beautifully with the acid fruits and berries. This dish is a surprise treat to the palate.

1 orange
1/4 C each of blackberries or
   strawberries or raspberries or
   all three

1 avocado (stone removed),
   sliced in half
pinch of freshly grated nutmeg

Chop and mix all fruits together. Fill the avocado boats with the fruit mixture and sprinkle with nutmeg. (Half an avocado is enough for one person.)

Pandora's Persimmon

This is one of the simplest recipes of all with fruit – and one of the most delicious.

2 very ripe persimmons
3/4 C desiccated coconut
a little spring water

5 ml (1 tsp) honey
5 ml (1 tsp) pure vanilla
   essence

Peel the ripe persimmons and blend thoroughly in a blender or food processor. Pour into chilled dishes. Mix the desiccated coconut in a blender with sufficient spring water to get the consistency of thick cream before adding the honey and vanilla essence and blending in well. Spoon the coconut cream on to the persimmon.

Live Apple Sauce

The quality and taste of this apple sauce depend entirely upon the quality of the apples themselves. If you make it with beautiful red apples it turns out to be a gorgeous pink colour. It is a real favourite for children and makes a lovely fruit breakfast or, served with 125 g (4 oz) chopped pecans, can be an excellent fruit meal for later on in the day.

4 apples, cored but not peeled and cut into small pieces
¾ C (more or less) of apple juice

dash of cinnamon or nutmeg or caraway or aniseed
a little raw honey (optional)

Liquefy the chopped apples in enough apple juice to make a medium-thick sauce. Add spices and a little raw honey to sweeten if desired. Serve immediately, lightly sprinkled with cinnamon, nutmeg, caraway or aniseed.

Almond Apple Porridge

Apples, with their remarkable ability to combine well with all sorts of foods which you wouldn't expect, make a wonderful marriage with almonds. Not a breakfast dish, because of the nuts it contains, this recipe nonetheless makes a yummy fruit meal for later on in the day.

4 apples, cored and cut into pieces but not peeled
¼ C finely chopped almonds

juice of 1 lemon
juice of 1 orange
sprinkling of nutmeg

Blend the apples with the other ingredients, keeping aside 5 ml (1 tsp) of the almonds and the nutmeg. When the mixture is fully blended, pour into four dishes and sprinkle with the remaining almonds and the nutmeg. Serve immediately.

Well Combined Mueslis

To encourage fat-loss it's best for the moment to steer clear of the traditional Birchermuesli because, for some, the combinations of milk products and grains – even though the grains have been soaked to break their sugars down into more simple ones – can be difficult to handle. Once you've lost all the extra fat you want to lose and your system has rebalanced itself, then you can indulge in the pleasures of the traditional Birchermuesli. Here are some suggestions:

Berry Muesli

150–225 g (5–7 oz) berries
(blueberries, strawberries,
blackberries, blackcurrants,
raspberries, etc.)
1 banana

15 ml (1 tbsp) finely chopped
almonds or pecans or
cashews
dash of cinnamon

Crush the berries with a fork. Slice the banana. Sprinkle with finely chopped almonds, pecans or cashews. Add a dash of cinnamon and serve immediately.

Other Mixed Fruit Muesli Suggestions

Blackberries and apples
Apples and sultanas
Apples and oranges
Apples and bananas

Plums, peaches and apricots
Strawberries and apples
Blueberries and apples

In each case remove the stones of any stoned fruit and blend in a food processor or chop finely with a knife. Otherwise the instructions are as for Berry Muesli.

Pear Surprise

A delicious fruit-and-nut dish. Not suitable for breakfast but excellent if you desire a fruit meal later on in the day.

4 pears, finely grated   *¼ C raw cashews, ground*

Fill four sorbet glasses with the finely grated pears and sprinkle each with the ground cashews. Serve immediately.

FRUIT DRINKS THAT MAKE A MEAL

Apricot Lhassi

A fresh fruit frappé with a delightful Eastern flavour.

*4–5 fresh apricots, stones
  removed*

*juice of 2 small oranges
pinch of coriander*

Put ingredients into blender and blend thoroughly. You may add ice if you wish to make a delicious cold summer breakfast.

Pineapple Blackberry Frappé

A fresh fruit frappé with a delightful Eastern flavour.

*2 C fresh pineapple chunks
1/2 C blackberries
juice of 1/2 a lime (optional)*

*spring or filtered water
  (optional)
ice cubes (optional)*

Place all the ingredients into a blender and liquidize. This can be thinned using a little spring or filtered water and chilled with an ice cube or two.

Strawberry Cream Shake

Not a breakfast recipe. This shake is a full fruit meal in itself and makes a lovely light supper for hot summer evenings.

*1/2 C fresh cashews
1 C spring or filtered water
1/2 C strawberries*

*15 ml (1 tbsp) raw honey
1/2 C fresh pineapple chunks
  (optional)*

Blend all the ingredients (including the pineapple chunks, if desired) in a food processor or blender and serve in a tall frosted glass. The quantities above make one very large shake.

Apple Raspberry Frappé

*2 sweet apples, cored but not
peeled, cut into small pieces
2.5 ml (1/2 tsp) finely chopped*

*lemon balm or mint
1/2 C fresh or frozen raspberries
spring or filtered water*

Place ingredients in blender and liquidize, adding a little spring or filtered water to thin it if you wish, and ice cubes if you want a chilled dish.

Banana-Coconut-Mint Frappé

Another full fruit meal that is rich and creamy.

2 very ripe bananas
¼ C desiccated or shredded
*   fresh coconut*

5 ml (1 tsp) freshly chopped
*   mint leaves*
ice cubes (optional)

Blend ingredients together in a food processor or blender and serve. You may add one or two ice cubes to chill.

Creamy Date Delight

2 very ripe bananas
4 fresh dates
15 ml (1 tbsp) shredded

coconut
½–1 C sparkling spring water

Blend the bananas, dates and coconut together thoroughly in a blender or food processor, then add the sparkling water and mix gently. Pour into chilled glasses and serve immediately.

Chapter Fifteen

Living Salads

To most people a salad is a pleasant side dish you use to set off the main course – which is usually meat-based. On the Raw Energy Food Combining Diet everything is turned around. All the salads you will find in this section are meals in their own right. They can be served on their own for lunch or dinner or they can be combined with protein or starch side-dishes – soups, cheeses, breads, grain dishes, fish, chicken, organic meat, egg dishes or game. They can also be made in much smaller quantities as side-salads to go with cooked main courses.

A living salad is one in which the main ingredients are drawn from sprouted seeds, grains and pulses. The other recipes are for salads based on fresh vegetables. And finally, of course, there are the crudités, which make wonderful starters for a meal or, served in greater quantity with a rich dip, dressing or seed cheese, can themselves become a beautiful meal.

The salads here are mostly quite elaborate and meant to be eaten as the centre of a meal. But you can also make some delightful simple salads by taking a root vegetable, such as a grated turnip, carrot or parsnip, and combining it in equal amounts with both a leafy vegetable, such as watercress, lamb's lettuce or Chinese leaf, and a bulb vegetable such as red or green pepper. This is the classic formula for the simple salad and it works every time served with a beautiful dressing (see pages 113-21 for recipes). It is hard to go wrong following this principle, so experiment for yourself.

Eat it Live

The living salad is the epitome of nutritional quality for encouraging fat-loss. It is made from the freshest and tastiest vegetables and sprouted seeds and grains that you can buy – or, far better, grow yourself. Make sure when you are choosing such things as cucumbers, celery and sweet peppers that they are firm and fresh and also that your carrots and broccoli are snappy and crisp.

Living salads can be made either by hand (in which case the vegetables are cut with a sharp knife or grated on a stainless-steel hand grater) or in a food processor. All the ingredients in a living salad are cut into bite-size pieces, except for lettuces and greens which are either broken into pieces or left in larger pieces in order to form a bed for the sprouts.

You can turn most of these salads into a protein meal by adding a protein-based dip or salad dressing. You can turn them into a starch meal by eating them with a good wholegrain bread – preferably rye or pumpernickel, since the gluten in wheat tends to clog the intestines and may interfere with the elimination process – or serving them with wholegrain (sugar-free) Scottish oatcakes, wholegrain crispbread or other wholegrain crackers.

You should treat the recipes listed below only as guidelines. The real pleasure of living cuisine is creating masterpieces of your own out of the simple things which you grow yourself on your windowsill or find in your refrigerator.

The Red Witch Salad (neutral)

The combination of radicchio with lamb's lettuce creates one of my favourite salads.

125 g (4 oz) radicchio
(Italian red lettuce) divided
into leaves
50 g (2 oz) lamb's lettuce
3 sticks of celery, chopped
2 large carrots, grated
1 C fresh mung-bean sprouts
75 g (3 oz) chicory, divided
into leaves
1 avocado, peeled and sliced
4 spring onions, chopped
finely

For the Dressing
15 ml (1 tbsp) virgin olive oil
15 ml (1 tbsp) lemon or lime
juice
5 ml (1 tsp) Meaux mustard
10 ml (2 tsp) chopped fresh
basil
black pepper

Keeping out eight radicchio leaves and five leaves of chicory, mix all the salad ingredients together in a bowl. Then mix the ingredients for the dressing together in a screw-top jar by shaking well. Pour the dressing over the salad and toss. Arrange the radicchio and chicory leaves which you have saved in a 'sunburst' around a platter. Serve the rest of the salad in the middle of the leaves.

Sprouted Lentil Salad (neutral)

This salad is a way of transforming the humble lentil into something quite marvellous.

1½ C fresh lentil sprouts
1 large red pepper (seeds
removed), diced
125 g (4 oz) broccoli florets
125 g (4 oz) cauliflower
florets
175 g (6 oz) button
mushrooms, sliced finely

For the Dressing
30 ml (2 tbsp) sesame oil
30 ml (2 tbsp) cider vinegar
15 ml (1 tbsp) freshly grated
root ginger
30 ml (2 tbsp) fresh orange
juice
5 ml (1 tsp) vegetable bouillon
powder or soy sauce

Mix the salad ingredients together in a large bowl. Mix the dressing ingredients together in a screw-top jar and shake well. Pour the dressing over the salad and toss. You may garnish this salad with ¼ C of sunflower seeds if you like; this turns it into a protein salad.

A Touch of the Orient (neutral)

This salad has a typically oriental flavour and feel to it. It is pleasant served with slivers of blanched almonds, in which case it turns into a protein meal.

1 C mung-bean sprouts
1 C fenugreek sprouts
1 C adzuki sprouts
1 yellow or red pepper, seeded and chopped
1 medium carrot, chopped into ½ in cubes
½ C Chinese leaves, shredded finely
30 ml (2 tbsp) chopped fresh parsley

2 cloves of garlic, chopped very finely
¼ C chopped spring onions
1 C spring or filtered water
juice of lemon
45 ml (3 tbsp) tamari
1 avocado, chopped into small cubes
the outside leaves of a cos lettuce

Marinate the sprouts and vegetables (except for the cos leaves and the avocado) in the water, to which you've added the lemon juice and tamari. Put in the refrigerator to chill. Then pour off the water and serve with small cubes of avocado on a bed of cos lettuce leaves, with or without a dressing.

Blue Dolphin Salad (neutral)

This simple living salad can be completely transformed in quality depending upon the kind of dressing you serve it with. Experiment with a seed cheese, a good mayonnaise or a light Italian herbal dressing to see which you like best.

1 C lentil sprouts
1 C fenugreek sprouts
1 C alfalfa sprouts
1 C Chinese leaves, shredded finely

3 carrots, sliced in paper-thin rounds
1 avocado, cubed
4 tomatoes, diced

Mix the ingredients together and toss with your favourite dressing. Serve immediately.

Spring Gardens Salad (neutral)

Another simple living salad, this dish goes particularly well with Racy Red Cheese dressing, Light Vinaigrette or Avocado Delight.

2 C radicchio, torn into small pieces	1 turnip, sliced thinly into matchsticks
1 C alfalfa sprouts	24 black olives, stoned
1 punnet of mustard and cress	4 tomatoes, sectioned into quarters
1 C thinly sliced cos lettuce	chives or herbs (optional)
2 small carrots, washed but not peeled, sliced thinly	

Put ingredients (except the tomatoes) into a large bowl and toss with salad dressing of your choice. Place tomato quarters around the side and sprinkle with some chopped chives or fresh herbs if you like.

Branton's Booster (protein)

This protein-based living salad is particularly good when you feel the need for something quite substantial, especially if you are doing a lot of exercise. Thanks to the fact that it contains sprouted sunflower seeds, this is a salad that really feels as if it sticks to your ribs.

1 C sprouted sunflower seeds	3 celery stalks, cut lengthways three or four times then chopped crossways finely
2 C chopped chicory	
2 C alfalfa sprouts	
1 C lentil sprouts or mung-bean sprouts	2 green peppers, seeded and chopped
5 tomatoes, sliced thinly	1½ C chopped fennel

Toss all the ingredients together and serve with Horsey Tomato Dressing or Light Vinaigrette.

Cress Special (neutral)

This is an ultra-light salad which contains no oil. The combination of lemon and tamari is quite delightful.

1 C curled cress, water cress or
    roquette
1 C alfalfa sprouts
1/2 C lentil sprouts
2 sticks of celery, cut
    lengthways three or four
    times then chopped
    crossways finely

1 avocado, peeled and cubed
45 ml (3 tbsp) tamari
1 clove of garlic, finely
    chopped
30 ml (2 tbsp) parsley or fresh
    basil, finely chopped
juice of 2 lemons

Toss the ingredients into a bowl, sprinkle with the lemon juice and tamari and serve.

The Green Light (neutral)

I like to serve this salad with Creamy Lemon Dressing.

1/2 C alfalfa sprouts
1/2 C mung-bean sprouts
1/2 C fenugreek sprouts
1/2 C sunflower-seed sprouts
1/2 C chicory, sliced finely
1/2 C cos lettuce
4 spring onions, chopped
    finely

4 tomatoes, chopped
1 courgette, sliced finely
2 stalks of celery, cut
    lengthways three or four
    times then chopped
    crossways finely
1 large beetroot, grated finely
2 large carrots, grated finely

Mix all the ingredients (except the grated carrots and beetroot) in a bowl and toss with salad dressing. Arrange the carrots and the beetroot separately around the rim to decorate. Serve immediately.

Crudités

One of my favourite hors d'oeuvres or salads is a platter of crudités – crunchy raw vegetables and fruit sliced or chopped so that you can pick the pieces up with your fingers. They can be eaten dipped into sauce (see pages 113-21) or simply sprinkled with a light dressing and a few toasted fennel or caraway seeds. The important thing is how you prepare them.

Sticks and Matchsticks

Make sticks from carrots, turnips, courgettes, cucumbers, celery and pineapple. To make matchsticks just keep chopping until you get 'baby sticks' that are about the size of a match (you can also make matchsticks from green and red peppers). To keep sticks fresh, put them into a bowl of cold water with a squeeze of lemon and refrigerate them.

Slices

Some vegetables are particularly nice sliced diagonally. This makes larger pieces for better 'dunkers'. Try diagonal slices of cucumber, carrot and white radish. Very thin slices of small beetroot, Jerusalem artichoke, kohlrabi and turnip are also nice. Large apples sliced crossways can be used as 'bread' for open-air sandwiches. Sweet peppers cut crossways make attractive rings. Try cutting ½ inch slices of peppers and placing around a bundle of carrot or celery sticks.

Whole Vegetables

Button mushrooms with their stalks on, whole baby carrots, the small centre stalks from a head of celery, whole young green beans that have been topped and tailed, florets of cauliflower, radishes, young spring onions – simply trimmed and rinsed, they all make great crudités.

Wedges

Wedges of tomato, chicory, Webb's Wonder lettuce, oranges, tangerines, apples and pears.

It is nice to garnish a plate of crudités with some half-slices of lemon, sprigs of watercress, parsley or mint and some of your favourite sprouts.

SUPERSALADS

Greek Delight Plus (protein)

A new twist on a classic Greek salad, with extra protein added in the form of feta cheese.

4 inch piece of cucumber
125–250 g (4–8 oz) feta
  cheese
250 g (8 oz) tomatoes
1 dozen black olives
3 C fresh alfalfa sprouts

For the Dressing
1 clove of garlic, chopped
  finely
45 ml (3 tbsp) chopped fresh
  basil
15 ml (1 tbsp) lemon juice
15 ml (1 tbsp) virgin olive oil
black pepper

Chop the cucumber, feta cheese and tomatoes into small pieces. Mix them in a bowl together with the black olives. Mix the dressing ingredients together in a screw-top jar by shaking them. Pour the dressing over the salad and toss. Then arrange on a bed of alfalfa sprouts and serve on a platter.

Spinach Splendour (protein)

This delicious complete-meal salad is set off by a subtle dressing based on dry white wine and walnut oil.

75 g (3 oz) spinach leaves
1½ C alfalfa sprouts
6 to 8 radishes, sliced finely
125 g (4 oz) mushrooms,
  sliced finely
4 hard-boiled eggs, either
  chopped finely or grated

For the Dressing
30 ml (2 tbsp) walnut oil
45 ml (3 tbsp) lemon juice

½ lemon rind grated
15 ml (1 tbsp) freshly grated
  root ginger
30 ml (2 tbsp) dry white wine
2 cloves of garlic, chopped
  finely
5 ml (1 tsp) vegetable bouillon
  powder or sea salt or soy
  sauce
black pepper

Wash the spinach leaves and dry them thoroughly in a spinner or in a towel. Combine all the ingredients of the salad together in a large bowl. Mix the ingredients of the dressing together by shaking well in a screw-top jar. Pour dressing over the salad and toss. Add the grated or chopped hard-boiled eggs to the top and serve chilled.

Scottish Pine (protein)

The combination of lamb's lettuce with pine kernels is unbeatable – another top favourite.

250 g (8 oz) tomatoes, diced
6 radishes, sliced finely
6 spring onions, chopped
finely
250 g (8 oz) lamb's lettuce
45 ml (3 tbsp) parsley,
chopped finely
1 C alfalfa or fenugreek
sprouts
75 g (3 oz) pine kernels

For the Dressing
15 ml (1 tbsp) cider vinegar
45 ml (3 tbsp) sunflower oil
1 clove of garlic, chopped
finely
5 ml (1 tsp) vegetable bouillon
powder or sea salt
5 ml (1 tsp) Meaux mustard
black pepper

Combine the finely chopped ingredients with the lamb's lettuce and the sprouts. Mix the dressing ingredients together in a screw-top bottle and shake well. Pour the dressing over the salad, toss, and garnish with the pine kernels. Serve chilled.

Celeriac Special (protein)

We've grown celeriac in our garden all winter. It is a pleasure to have this crunchy, delicately flavoured organic root as part of almost any salad.

4 medium celeriac, grated
finely
2 medium carrots, scrubbed
but not peeled, grated finely
125 g (4 oz) chopped pecans
10 chives, leaves chopped very
finely
½ red pepper, seeded and
chopped finely

½ green pepper, seeded and
chopped finely
mayonnaise for dressing (see
pages 113-16)
12 black olives, stones
removed
outer leaves from a head of
radicchio or chicory

Mix all the ingredients except the olives and the leaves together, dressed with a good mayonnaise. Arrange on a bed of chicory or radicchio leaves, decorate with the olives, and serve immediately.

Raita (protein)

A delicious cucumber salad which can be made with a low-fat dairy yogurt.

3 finely diced carrots
handful of fresh peas
1 large cucumber, sliced
lengthways, then crossways,
in order to produce slivers
each about 1½–2 inches
long

1 C low-fat yogurt
juice of 1 lemon
30 ml (2 tbsp) fresh mint
leaves, finely chopped
crisp salad greens

Make sure the carrots, peas and cucumber are chilled thoroughly. Take a little yogurt to which you have added the finely chopped fresh mint leaves and the lemon juice and pour over the salad, mixing well. Serve on crisp salad greens.

Devil's Delight (neutral)

Raw beetroot has remarkable properties for detoxification; it's also an excellent source of vitamin C and a number of important minerals. And it is delicious – particularly married with fresh apples. Once you taste it you will wonder how you could ever eat this beautiful red root vegetable cooked.

3 raw beetroot
3 green apples
3 white radishes

For the Dressing
30 ml (2 tbsp) sunflower oil
15 ml (1 tbsp) lemon juice

5 ml (1 tsp) Meaux mustard
45 ml (3 tbsp) chopped parsley
4 spring onions, chopped
finely ground black pepper
5 ml (1 tsp) vegetable bouillon
powder

Grate the beetroot, apples and radishes, preferably in a food processor, then mix together in a bowl. Put the dressing ingredients in a screw-top jar and shake. Pour your dressing over the salad and toss.

Green Glory (neutral)

This is a delightful, crunchy summer salad which goes equally well garnished with chopped eggs as a protein meal, or served with a baked potato or a starchy soup as a starch meal.

250 g (8 oz) Chinese leaves,
  shredded finely
1 green pepper (seeds
  removed), chopped
45 ml (3 tbsp) lovage leaves,
  chopped finely or fresh
  mint, chopped finely
4 sticks of celery, cut
  lengthways three or four
  times, then chopped
  crossways finely
3 spring onions, sliced
  diagonally

For the Dressing
60 ml (4 tbsp) mayonnaise
30 ml (2 tbsp) orange juice
grated rind from ½ orange
30 ml (2 tbsp) chopped parsley
5 ml (1 tsp) vegetable bouillon
  powder or sea salt
2 cloves of garlic, chopped
  finely

Shred, chop and prepare the vegetables and put them into a large bowl. Mix dressing ingredients in a screw-top jar and shake well. Pour the dressing over the salad and toss. Garnish with lovage leaves or fresh mint. Serve chilled.

Tomato Treasures (neutral)

This stuffed tomato salad is delicious and so pretty to serve.

8 tomatoes
1 avocado, peeled and stoned
juice of 2 lemons
2 cloves of garlic, crushed
45 ml (3 tbsp) finely chopped
  basil
dash of Tabasco sauce to taste
5 ml (1 tsp) vegetable bouillon
  powder or sea salt
2 C fresh alfalfa sprouts
50 g (2 oz) lamb's lettuce
6 spring onions, chopped
  diagonally

For the Dressing
15 ml (1 tbsp) olive oil
15 ml (1 tbsp) lemon juice
45 ml (3 tbsp) chopped fresh
  parsley
5 ml (1 tsp) vegetable bouillon
  powder
1 clove of garlic, chopped
  finely
15 ml (1 tbsp) chopped fresh
  basil
black pepper (optional)

Slice the lid from each tomato and remove the insides with a spoon. Mix the insides in a blender or food processor with all the other ingredients except the alfalfa sprouts, the lamb's lettuce and the spring onions; then spoon back into the tomato shells. Toss the salad made out of the alfalfa sprouts, lamb's lettuce and spring onions with the dressing, and season with black pepper if desired. Spread on to a platter and place the tomatoes on top. Serve chilled.

Jerusalem Artichoke Salad (neutral)

A sweet and crunchy winter salad, this dish is another favourite. It is simple to prepare but tastes like something very special.

6 Jerusalem artichokes, grated
 finely
3 carrots, grated finely
1 apple, chopped finely
45 ml (3 tbsp) parsley,
 chopped finely
3 stalks of celery, cut
 lengthways two or three
 times then chopped
 crossways finely

¾ C Chinese leaves, chopped
 finely

For the Dressing
mayonnaise (see pages 113-
 16)
cayenne pepper
garlic

Mix together and serve with the dressing. You can turn this salad into an excellent protein salad by sprinkling some pumpkin or sunflower seeds over the top.

Watercress Salad (neutral)

This is a special treat for me because I love the slightly bitter taste and the beautiful dark green colour of fresh watercress.

3 C cos lettuce, torn into small
 pieces
1 bunch of watercress, cut into
 ½ inch lengths
4 spring onions, chopped
 finely

¾ C courgettes, grated
2 carrots, grated
4 tomatoes, quartered
45–60 ml (3–4 tbsp)
 sunflower seeds (optional)

Combine all the ingredients and serve with a vinaigrette (see page 117). This salad can be turned into a beautiful protein dish by sprinkling 45–60 ml (3–4 tbsp) of sunflower seeds on the top.

Root-is-Best Salad (neutral)

This shows how delicious the root vegetable can be.

2 turnips, grated finely
3 fresh parsnips, scrubbed but not peeled, and grated
2 carrots, scrubbed but not peeled, and grated
1 sweet potato, peeled and grated or 1 potato, grated
3 spring onions, chopped finely
1/2 red pepper, deseeded and chopped finely
1/2 green pepper, deseeded and chopped finely
15 ml (1 tbsp) chopped summer savory or lovage
juice of 1 lemon
2 C Chinese leaves, or lettuce, finely grated or chopped
mayonnaise (see pages 113-16)
spring or filtered water

Mix all vegetable ingredients except the Chinese leaves and pour lemon juice over them. Toss well and serve on a bed of finely grated Chinese leaves or lettuce with a good mayonnaise which has been thinned with a little spring or filtered water.

Bulgar Salad with Endive (starch)

A delicious and substantial dish which, thanks to the endive and the bulgar wheat, is high in vitamin E. The contrast between the rich graininess of the Bulgar wheat and the delicate flavour of the endive is most pleasing.

125 g (4 oz) bulgar wheat
1 endive
6 spring onions
a punnet of salad cress

For the Dressing
15 ml (1 tbsp) sunflower oil
15 ml (3 tsp) chopped fresh parsley

juice of 1/2 lemon
rind of 1/2 lemon
5 ml (1 tsp) white-wine vinegar
1 tsp vegetable bouillon powder or sea salt
black pepper
1 clove of garlic, chopped finely

Soak the bulgar wheat overnight or for at least three hours in enough water to cover. Then drain excess water. Put dressing ingredients in a screw-top jar and mix by shaking well. Add endive, onions and salad cress to the bulgar wheat in a bowl and mix. Pour the dressing over the salad and toss.

Celebration Salad (starch)

This main-dish salad is another beautiful marriage between vegetable and grain, set off by the delicate flavour of sesame oil, lemon and orange which go into the dressing.

175 g (6 oz) long-grain brown rice
3 large carrots, sliced in very thin discs
1 C fenugreek sprouts
¼ cucumber, sliced finely
125 g (4 oz) garden peas
black pepper
1 ml (¼ tsp) vegetable bouillon powder
a few sprigs of mint or lovage

For the Dressing
juice of ½ lemon
juice of ½ orange
10 ml (2 tsp) sesame oil
2.5 ml (½ tsp) grated or ground nutmeg
30 ml (2 tbsp) finely chopped fresh mint

Put the rice into a saucepan. Cover with about 2 inches of water, bring to the boil and simmer for 35 minutes or until tender. Put the dressing ingredients together and shake in a screw-top jar. Pour over the rice while it is still warm and combine carefully. Let the mixture cool completely. Add the vegetables to the rice. Season with a little black pepper and vegetable bouillon powder, garnish with mint or lovage.

Potato Supreme (starch)

This is a light and delicately flavoured potato salad, very different from the stodgy, oily variety which most people know.

450 g (1 lb) potatoes,
preferably organic
½ cucumber, diced
5 sticks of celery, diced
2 large carrots, diced
3 spring onions, diced
45 ml (3 tbsp) finely chopped
fresh parsley
2 cloves of garlic, chopped
finely
5 ml (1 tsp) dill, chopped
finely

For the Dressing
75 ml (5 tbsp) mayonnaise
(see pages 113-14)
30 ml (2 tbsp) lemon juice
5 ml (1 tsp) Meaux mustard
5 ml (1 tsp) vegetable bouillon
powder or soy sauce
black pepper

Scrub the potatoes carefully but do not peel. Add them to a saucepan of boiling water and simmer for 15 to 20 minutes until they are tender. Drain and cool, then dice. Mix the ingredients of the dressing together with a spoon and add to the potatoes. Now chill and when completely chilled add the remaining ingredients and serve.

Chapter Sixteen

You're the Tops

The fresh vegetables, herbs and other delicacies that you put into a salad are only half the story: the other half is the dressing. So splendid are some of the dressings that you can use on the Raw Energy Food Combining Diet that they will undoubtedly delight your family and friends while at the same time helping you trim away the excess fat.

Dressings come in two varieties: they can be protein in nature, like some of the lovely seed dressings and sunflower creams, or they can be neutral (and used on either protein or starch salads) as is the usual Italian or French dressing to which most people are accustomed.

So filling are some of the protein dressings that they are all the extra protein for a meal which you will need when served with a large delicious salad. Many recipes can be for either a dip or a dressing, depending upon how thick you make them. The dips are best used for crudités; the dressings are best poured over salads which have been grated or chopped or over sprouts.

Mayonnaise (protein)

This is a classic mayonnaise which can be varied by adding different herbs, Dijon mustard, curry powder or garlic to it, depending upon the use to which you want to put it.

2 raw egg yolks at room temperature	*2 C salad oil (this can be a mixture of olive oil with*
5 ml (1 tsp) dry mustard	*sesame or sunflower oil or,*
dash of cayenne	*for a light dressing, it can*
5 ml (1 tsp) vegetable bouillon powder	*be entirely sunflower or corn oil)*
juice of 1 lemon	

In a food processor or blender, thoroughly blend the egg yolks with the mustard, the cayenne and the vegetable bouillon powder. Add 30 ml (2 tbsp) of lemon juice. While still blending add the oil, a few drops at a time, very slowly until about half the oil has been blended. Finally, beat in the remaining oil, about two tablespoons at a time. This will keep in the refrigerator for five to six days.

Sunny Tomato Special (protein)

A surprising combination of the tangy flavour of tomatoes with the richness of fresh sunflower seeds.

6 fresh tomatoes or 1 tin of tomatoes	*juice of 2 lemons*
1 C sunflower seeds	*15 ml (1 tbsp) fresh finely chopped parsley or fresh*
5 ml (1 tsp) vegetable bouillon powder or soy sauce	*basil (if you can't get the fresh herbs you may use*
1 clove of garlic, finely chopped	*much smaller quantities of the dried ones)*

Put the ingredients together in a blender or food processor and blend thoroughly. If you want a thicker consistency add more sunflower seeds (but remember the dressing will thicken as it stands); if you want a thinner consistency add a little water. Chill thoroughly before use. Made with fresh tomatoes this will keep for two days in the refrigerator; made with tinned tomatoes it will keep for four or five.

Nut Mayonnaise (protein)

A delicious alternative mayonnaise which goes beautifully with crudités and also as a garnish for lightly steamed vegetables.

125 g (4 oz) cashews
1 C spring water
2 cloves of garlic, finely
    chopped
juice of 1 lemon

5 ml (1 tsp) vegetable
    bouillon, or sea salt or soy
    sauce
spring onions, finely chopped

Blend together well in a food processor or blender, chill and serve. This recipe will keep for four or five days covered in the refrigerator.

Soya Cottage Cheese (protein)

Light, high in protein, low in fat and simply yummy.

2 C soybean curd
¾ C nut mayonnaise or
    tahini mayonnaise or
    plain mayonnaise
5 ml (1 tsp) vegetable bouillon
    powder or soy sauce or sea
    salt
5 ml (1 tsp) caraway seeds

5 ml (1 tsp) mild curry powder
1 clove of garlic, chopped
    finely
handful of fresh herbs (mint,
    lovage, lemon balm) if
    available
30 ml (2 tbsp) chopped chives

Mash the soybean curd well with a fork, add the other ingredients and blend. Chill before serving. This dressing will keep up to a week in the refrigerator.

Raw Houmus (protein)

2 C sprouted chickpeas
    (sprouted for two to three
    days)
1 clove of garlic, chopped
    finely
45 ml (3 tbsp) tahini
juice of 3 lemons

enough water to thin
5 ml (1 tsp) vegetable bouillon
    powder or 10 ml (2 tsp) soy
    sauce
15 ml (3 tsp) chopped spring
onions or chives

Put ingredients (except chives or spring onions) into a food processor or blender and blend thoroughly. Then mix in chopped chives or spring onions and chill. This dressing will keep for two to three days in the refrigerator.

Extralite Tahini Mayonnaise (protein)

This mayonnaise makes a delicious dip for crudités.
Warning: it's *very* rich.

1 C tahini
1 C water
1 clove of garlic, finely
  chopped
30 ml (2 tbsp) chopped fresh
  parsley

5 ml (1 tsp) vegetable bouillon
  powder
juice of 3 lemons

Put ingredients into a blender or food processor or mix
them together by hand until you get a smooth consistency.
Refrigerate. This dressing will keep up to a week in the
refrigerator.

Tahini Mayonnaise (protein)

This mayonnaise is also delicious as a dip for crudités or
served over steamed vegetables.

juice of 2 lemons or ¼ C cider
  vinegar
2.5 ml (½ tsp) vegetable
  bouillon powder or soy
  sauce

60 ml (4 tbsp) tahini
½ C water
1 clove of chopped garlic
¼ C olive oil

Mix all ingredients except olive oil in blender or food
processor until thoroughly blended. Add olive oil very
slowly, as much as you need to thicken. Store in glass jar in
refrigerator. Will keep for four to five days.

Sprout Splendour (protein)

1 C alfalfa sprouts
4 sprigs of celery, chopped very
  finely
5 ml (1 tsp) vegetable bouillon
  powder or 30 ml (2 tbsp)
  tamari

¾ C sunflower oil
juice of 2 lemons
15 ml (1 tbsp) finely chopped
  onion
15 ml (1 tbsp) sesame seeds
5 ml (1 tsp) Dijon mustard

Blend thoroughly and serve on a fresh green salad or use as
a dip. Must be eaten same day – does not keep well.

Light Vinaigrette (neutral)

30 ml (2 tbsp) cider vinegar
60 ml (4 tbsp) sesame oil
2.5 ml (½ tsp) Meaux
 mustard

2.5 ml (½ tsp) tarragon
2.5 ml (½ tsp) chervil
2.5 ml (½ tsp) vegetable
 bouillon powder or sea salt

Mix the vinegar, oil, mustard, herbs and bouillon powder or salt together and blend well by putting them all into a jar with a screw-top lid and shaking thoroughly.

Celery Special (neutral)

This is a surprisingly fresh and unusually flavoured dressing which goes well with an all-green salad. I particularly like it with lamb's lettuce.

½ C olive oil
¼ C celery seeds
3 spring onions, chopped
 finely
1 clove of garlic, chopped
 finely

2.5 ml (½ tsp) marjoram
10 ml (2 tsp) fresh parsley,
 chopped finely
5 ml (1 tsp) vegetable bouillon
 powder or a little sea salt

Blend well by shaking in a screw-top jar.

Horsey Tomato Dressing (neutral)

This is a delightful dressing to serve over finely sliced cucumbers in summertime.

½ C olive oil
juice from 2 lemons
2.5 ml (½ tsp) Dijon mustard
10 ml (2 tsp) horseradish
1 clove of garlic, crushed

2 fresh tomatoes
2.5 ml (½ tsp) sesame seeds
5 ml (1 tsp) vegetable bouillon
 powder or other seasoning

Blend well in a blender or food processor and serve chilled.

Parsley Cream (protein)

This is a low-fat salad dressing based on yogurt. It's particularly good served on salads of sprouts, cucumbers and tomatoes. It also makes a nice addition to a slaw.

117

1 C natural low-fat yogurt
juice of 1 lemon
2.5 ml (½ tsp) dill
small onion, chopped

10 ml (2 tsp) chopped parsley
2.5 ml (½ tsp) vegetable
bouillon powder or soy
sauce

Blend well together by hand or in a blender. Will keep four to five days in a refrigerator.

Pink Yogurt Dressing (protein)

Not as good as pink champagne, perhaps, but sheer delight on sprouts and cucumber.

1 C thick yogurt
60 ml (4 tbsp) tomato purée
5 ml (1 tsp) Meaux mustard
½ clove garlic, chopped finely

2.5 ml (½ tsp) vegetable
bouillon powder
15 ml (1 tbsp) chopped
shallots or spring onions

Mix everything but the shallots together well – in a blender, if possible. Then add the shallots and finish mixing. Serve chilled. Will keep up to five days in the refrigerator.

Green Dream (protein)

This dressing is ideal for a potato salad. It's also delicious on finely sliced tomatoes.

2 cucumbers
3 spring onions, chopped
  finely
juice of 1 lemon
5 ml (1 tsp) horseradish

2.5 ml (½ tsp) vegetable
bouillon powder or soy
sauce or sea salt1 C
natural yogurt, or home
made mayonnaise

Blend together in food processor all ingredients except mayonnaise, or yogurt. Fold into the mayonnaise or yogurt and chill. Will not keep for more than a day.

Avocado Delight (neutral)

This is a superb dip or dressing, and very rich indeed. Excellent on a sprout salad or as a dip for crudités.

1 avocado, peeled and stoned
juice of 1 lemon
juice of ½ orange
1 small onion, chopped finely
1 clove of garlic, chopped
   finely

handful of fresh herbs – mint,
   parsley or basil
Black pepper

Blend all the ingredients in a food processor or blender and serve. This dip will not keep for more than one day in a refrigerator.

Creamy Lemon Dressing (protein)

juice of 2 lemons
30 ml (2 tbsp) chopped
   cashews

2.5 ml (½ tsp) vegetable
   bouillon powder
½ C sunflower oil

Combine ingredients (except the oil) together in a blender or food processor and blend thoroughly. Then add the oil slowly, drop by drop.

French Spice (neutral)

A pleasant light dressing that seems to complement any salad.

juice of 2 lemons
2 ripe tomatoes
1 clove of garlic
12 chives, chopped finely
5 ml (1 tsp) powdered kelp
   (optional)

⅓ C sunflower oil
5 ml (1 tsp) cayenne
15 ml (1tbsp) tamari
15 ml (1 tbsp) Dijon mustard
5 ml (1 tsp) vegetable bouillon
   powder

Blend ingredients together in a food processor or blender until thoroughly mixed. This dressing may be refrigerated and kept for up to four days.

Italian Dressing (neutral)

Another classic dressing. It also goes well with my favourite greens, such as, lamb's lettuce, roquette, American land cress and curly cress served on their own and sprinkled with parsley.

1 pint virgin olive oil
30 ml (2 tbsp) paprika
30 ml (2 tbsp) finely chopped
  fresh basil
10 ml (2 tsp) vegetable
  bouillon powder or 30 ml
  (2 tbsp) of tahini

2.5 ml (½ tsp) dried oregano
pinch of cayenne
pinch of kelp (optional)
¼ C chopped fennel
2.5 ml (½ tsp) finely chopped
  red pepper

Put ingredients into a screw-top jar and shake vigorously until well mixed. You may thin this dressing with water if it seems too thick. It will keep well for up to 10 days in the refrigerator.

Wild Carrot Dressing (protein)

This dressing is one of my favourites. It goes well either on a salad or on steamed vegetables.

3 large carrots, washed and
  cut into small pieces
10 chives, chopped finely
5 ml (1 tsp) vegetable bouillon
  powder

1 C of blanched almonds
  (preferably soaked overnight
  in 1–2 C of spring or
  filtered water)
10 ml (2 tsp) chopped parsley

Put all ingredients into a food processor or blender and blend with as much water as you need to make the dressing the consistency you want. It's best to leave it thick if you want to use it as a dip, or make it thinner as a dressing to pour over salads.

Green Glory Dressing (protein)

This dressing is an absolute cinch to make if you have fresh herbs in the garden; you may be amazed to find how many herbs and of what different varieties you can use to make it.

30 ml (2 tbsp) virgin olive oil
30 ml (2 tbsp) lemon juice
¾ C fresh natural yogurt
30–120 ml (2–8 tbsp) fresh
  herbs from the garden

(whatever you have
available: lovage, mint,
apple mint, lemon mint,
balm, chives, spring
onions, etc.)

Place all the ingredients in blender or food processor and blend thoroughly until the dressing turns green. This dressing will keep for four to five days in the refrigerator.

Racy Red Cheese (protein)

This delicious dip or dressing can be served with crudités, over a salad or added to freshly steamed or wok-fried vegetables. It's a beautiful pink colour and has a refreshing zippy taste.

1 C cashews or *pine nuts*
1 C filtered or *spring water*
5 ml (1 tsp) vegetable bouillon powder or *sea salt*
2.5 ml ($\frac{1}{2}$ tsp) caraway seeds

juice of 2 lemons
$\frac{1}{2}$ C pimentos
4 chopped spring onions or *chives*

Mix all the ingredients (except the chives or spring onions) in a blender or food processor until smooth. Blend in the chives or spring onions by hand and serve. This dip may be kept in the refrigerator for four to five days.

Chapter Seventeen

Peasant Soups

There was a time when a good soup formed the basis of a main meal for the whole family – and in many parts of the world it still does. I often use the heartier full-bodied soups in this way, particularly in winter. I take whatever vegetables I can find in the garden or in the refrigerator, chop them and put them into a big pot with fresh or dried herbs and perhaps a cereal such as millet, barley, rice or buckwheat. The results are wonderful – particularly if you use vegetable bouillon as your stock. Once you get the hang of it you simply can't help but make a good soup.

The soups in this section fall into two categories – those which are living and therefore either served cold or heated to no more than about 110°F (43°C) in order to preserve the enzymes they contain, and the traditional old-fashioned soups which most of our ancestors lived on. Try both types – as main dishes and as side dishes to go with total-meal salads. I hope you'll like them as much as I and my family do.

Leek and Potato Soup (starch)
This is a delicious and creamy soup which goes beautifully with a neutral salad to make up a whole meal. It is a starch soup.

1 large onion, sliced
3 medium-sized leeks, sliced
　　lengthwise, washed and
　　chopped into fine pieces
3 large potatoes, peeled and
　　sliced
15 ml (1 tbsp) olive oil

¾ pint spring or filtered water
　　(more if needed)
10 ml (2 tsp) vegetable
　　bouillon powder
2.5 ml (½ tsp) freshly grated
　　nutmeg or ground pepper

Brown the onion, leeks and potatoes in the olive oil for ten minutes until onion becomes translucent. Boil the water in a kettle and pour over the browned vegetables. Bring to the boil, add the vegetable powder, and simmer for 10–15 minutes. Liquidize in a food processor or blender and serve hot with grated nutmeg (or ground pepper if preferred) sprinkled on top of each bowl.

Barley Mushroom Soup (starch)

A starch soup, this is a beautiful winter meal which is welcoming, warming and friendly. The ideal thing for a cosy winter evening in front of the fire.

½ C barley
2 pints spring or filtered water
45 ml (3 tbsp) olive oil
3 cloves of garlic, minced
2 large onions, chopped finely
450 g (1 lb) fresh mushrooms,
　　sliced thinly

15 ml (3 tsp) vegetable
　　bouillon powder
1 avocado
½ C dry white wine
freshly ground black pepper

Cook the barley in half of the water until tender, then add the remaining water. In another pan, sauté the garlic and the onions in the olive oil; when they are softened, add the mushrooms. When everything is tender add to the barley and cook for another 35 minutes. Add the bouillon powder. Mash the avocado with a fork or blend in a blender or food processor and stir into the soup with the dry white wine just before serving. Add a generous grinding of black pepper.

Curried Pumpkin Soup (starch)

This starch soup is charming and spicy and goes beautifully with a sprout salad.

*2 medium onions, chopped
   finely
1 clove of garlic, chopped
   finely
2 C of fresh pumpkin, cut into
   small cubes (substitute
   marrow for this if you wish)
30 ml (2 tbsp) olive oil
3 C water or stock
250 g (½ lb) mushrooms,
   sliced*

*2.5 ml (½ tsp) ground cumin
2.5 ml (½ tsp) coriander
2.5 ml (½ tsp) cinnamon
2.5 ml (½ tsp) ground ginger
2.5 ml (½ tsp) dry mustard
10 ml (2 tsp) vegetable
   bouillon powder or sea salt
pinch of cayenne
juice of 2 fresh lemons*

Sauté the onions, the garlic, the pumpkin and the mushrooms in olive oil until soft. Add the boiled water and cook for 10 minutes. Add seasonings and cook for another five to ten minutes. Place in a blender or food processor and blend thoroughly. Add freshly squeezed lemon juice and serve.

Bioactive Avocado and Tomato (neutral)

This neutral soup is light and spicy. You can serve it hot or cold.

*8 ripe tomatoes
1 ripe avocado
2 spring onions, chopped
   finely
1 ml (¼ tsp) ground dill seed
pinch of cayenne*

*1 C spring or filtered water
10 ml (2 tsp) vegetable
   bouillon powder
5 ml (1 tsp) kelp (optional)
1 green pepper, chopped finely*

Blend all ingredients (except the finely chopped green pepper and two of the tomatoes) in a blender or food processor. Heat gently to warm but not above 115°F (46°C). Chop the last two tomatoes and add with the green pepper when you serve.

Chilled Cucumber Soup (protein)

This delightful protein soup 'can't be beat' on a hot summer day.

1 large cucumber
2 C natural yogurt
60 ml (4 tbsp) finely chopped mint
10 ml (2 tsp) vegetable bouillon powder

1 ml (¼ tsp) crushed poppy seed (optional)
ice (optional)

Chop cucumber and blend in blender or food processor with chilled yogurt. You may add a few cubes of ice to make it colder if you wish. After blending for two minutes, add vegetable bouillon powder and continue to blend with ice. Finally, add chopped mint and blend again very briefly. Pour into bowls and serve immediately with a little chopped mint or crushed poppy seed sprinkled on top.

Gazpacho (neutral)

Another delicious cold neutral summer soup which you can make as spicy as you like.

6 ripe tomatoes, chopped
½ cucumber, chopped
juice of 1 lemon
10 ml (2 tsp) vegetable bouillon powder
5 ml (1 tsp) kelp (optional)
1 clove garlic, finely chopped
½ red pepper, finely chopped

½ green pepper, finely chopped
4 spring onions, finely chopped
45 ml (3 tbsp) parsley, finely chopped
cayenne pepper to taste

Keeping aside a small portion of the tomatoes and of the chopped cucumber, put the rest of the tomatoes and cucumber, the lemon juice, bouillon powder, kelp (if desired) and garlic in a food processor or blender and liquidize. Add the peppers, spring onions and parsley and mix well, season to taste with cayenne pepper and serve with the tomatoes and cucumber you have kept aside.

Corn Soup (starch)

A starch dish, this soup is uncooked and can either be served cold or warm.

2 fresh ears of corn
300 ml (½ pint) warm spring
or filtered water
2 spring onions, chopped
5 ml (1 tsp) vegetable bouillon
powder
15 ml (1 tbsp) olive oil

¼ red pepper, chopped
¼ green pepper, chopped
15 ml (1 tbsp) watercress,
chopped finely
15 ml (1 tbsp) tahini
(optional)

Wash the corn and cut the kernels off the cob with a knife. Mix together with the water, spring onions, olive oil and vegetable bouillon powder, season with tahini (if desired), and blend until creamy in a blender or food processor. Add chopped peppers and watercress to each portion.

Raw Asparagus Soup (protein)

A very special uncooked but heated protein soup, this dish is a delicate marriage of the unusual taste and aroma of the asparagus with the rich sensuous quality of the cashews.

¾ C cashew nuts
3 C spring or filtered water
1 bunch fresh raw asparagus
(tips only)
3 sticks celery

10 ml (2 tsp) vegetable
bouillon powder
30 ml (2 tbsp) fresh lovage,
chopped finely (optional)
30 ml (2 tbsp) minced parsley

Place cashew nuts in food processor with 1°C hot water and blend thoroughly until they have been reduced to a cream. Add to the mixture the other ingredients, saving out the chopped parsley. Heat thoroughly but do not boil. Serve with sprinkling of parsley.

Scottish Barley Soup (starch)

Another starch dish, this is one of my favourite hearty soups. I like it best on chilly autumn evenings. It goes beautifully well with a mixed green salad full of fresh herbs.

1 C barley

1 litre (1¾ pints) spring or
   filtered water

2 onions chopped

3 carrots, chopped into cubes

6 sticks of celery, diced

125 g (4 oz) mushrooms,
   chopped (optional)

15 ml (1 tbsp) olive oil

1 tin tomatoes or 6 fresh
   tomatoes

3 cloves of garlic, chopped
   finely

30 ml (2 tbsp) parsley,
   chopped finely

Cook the barley for an hour in the water. In a separate pan, fry the onions, carrots, celery and (if you like) mushrooms in the olive oil. Add to the barley along with the tomatoes and garlic and simmer for 20 minutes. Serve piping hot, sprinkled with fresh parsley. If you prefer a smooth soup, liquidize it in a blender or food processor.

Seductive Celery Cream (protein)

I find this protein soup utterly irresistible, but then I have a special passion for cashews, whose creamy qualities help them marry well with crunchy celery.

1 litre (1¾ pints) spring or
   filtered water

½ C celery leaves and tops,
   chopped

¾ C cashews

1 medium onion, chopped
   finely

2 C chopped celery bottoms

2 medium carrots, diced

1 C fresh or frozen peas
   (optional)

15 ml (1 tbsp) olive oil

15 ml (3 tsp) vegetable
   bouillon powder or other
   seasoning

Put into blender half the water, celery tops and leaves and cashews and blend thoroughly. Meanwhile, sauté the onion, celery bottoms, the carrots and peas in the olive oil. Then add together with the vegetable bouillon powder, bring to the boil with the remainder of the water, and simmer for no more than 10 minutes. Serve warm.

High Potassium Broth (starch)

This is an excellent dish to use not only as a soup but also as a broth to drink if you wish to miss a meal or even a whole day's meals, or just as a substitute for tea or coffee during the day. To use the soup as a broth you discard the vegetables. As a soup you drink it vegetables and all. This broth makes an excellent bouillon to use in other soups.

4 medium potatoes (including
   skins), diced
4 finely diced carrots
3 finely diced celery sticks
2 C green peas
1 large onion, chopped
2 cloves garlic, crushed
discarded leaves from lettuce,
   cabbage, cauliflower,
   Brussels sprouts, etc.

1 tbsp vegetable bouillon
   powder
2 litres (3½ pints) spring or
   filtered water
45 ml (3 tbsp) fresh parsley,
   finely chopped

Clean and chop the leaves and vegetables, discarding any wilted parts, and put into the pot with all the other ingredients. Bring to the boil and let simmer for two hours, then strain. Garnish with chopped parsley and serve.

Garlic Soup (starch)

This starch soup is for garlic lovers only. My daughter Susannah and I constantly fight over how much garlic should go into soups, salads, sauces and other dishes. I am an enormous garlic fan; Susannah believes that one whiff of garlic is enough to keep her intoxicated for a week. This soup is definitely of my own devising: it is also absolutely delicious. Susannah, alas, has never tasted it. The mere sight of the recipe would make her cringe.

3 potatoes (with skins on)
2 carrots
3 sticks of celery
1 large onion
1 litre spring or filtered water
2 large heads garlic
pinch of oregano

2.5 ml (½ tsp) thyme
pinch of sage
dash of cayenne
30 ml (2 tbsp) fresh parsley,
   finely chopped
15 ml (1 tbsp) vegetable
   bouillon powder

Cut potatoes, carrots, celery and onion into cubes and add to water that has been brought to the boil. Break garlic into individual cloves and add these together with the herbs and spices. Add bouillon powder and bring to the boil; simmer for 20 to 30 minutes. Put soup into a blender or food processor and blend, or strain vegetables from it and serve as a clear broth with parsley sprinkled on top.

Courgette Tomato (neutral)

This neutral soup is beautifully light with a delicate Italian flavour to it.

3 medium courgettes, diced
3 sticks of celery, chopped
  finely
4 spring onions, chopped
1 large carrot, diced
1 clove of garlic, crushed or
  chopped
15 ml (1 tbsp) olive oil

6 tomatoes, peeled and
  chopped
15 ml (1 tbsp) fresh basil,
  chopped finely or 2.5 ml
  (½ tsp) oregano
15 ml (3 tsp) vegetable
  bouillon powder or other
  seasoning

Sauté all the vegetables (except the tomatoes) and garlic in the olive oil for five minutes. Then add the tomatoes and pour in enough boiling water to cover. Bring to the boil and simmer for 20–30 minutes. Serve sprinkled with fresh basil or oregano and season according to taste.

Split-Pea Soup (starch)

Another hearty starch soup which goes well with a green salad.

1 C dried split peas which
  have been soaked in water
  to cover overnight
1 large onion, chopped
2 medium carrots, diced
2 sticks of celery, diced
1 litre (1¾ pints) spring or
  filtered water

15 ml (1 tbsp) vegetable
  bouillon powder
30 ml (2 tbsp) chopped fresh
  herbs as available (parsley,
  lovage, sage, pot marjoram)

After the peas have been washed and soaked overnight, put them in a pot with all the vegetables and cover with water. Bring to the boil and simmer for 1½ hours until the peas are tender. Add the vegetable bouillon and fresh herbs five minutes before serving. If you want a smooth soup, put into a food processor or blender; otherwise serve as is.

Chapter Eighteen

Hot Veggies

Cooked vegetables have a marvellous flavour of their own – there's nothing like the crunchy pleasure of a baked potato stuffed with a well dressed living salad, the light crisp taste of stir-fried mange-tout spiked with almond slivers, or the spicy tang of a good curry. Each vegetable has its own character and, like a special child, needs to be handled in an individual way to get the most from it.

In this section you will find all sorts of vegetable dishes prepared in many different ways. Some are best used as small side-dishes; others – particularly some of the mixtures – make wonderful meals in themselves and are great for entertaining.

Super Stir-Fries

These attractive and quick vegetable dishes are based on the Chinese principle of frying vegetables very quickly in a minute quantity of light oil. If you're in a hurry, all of your vegetables may be prepared in advance, chopped and left in the refrigerator for when you are ready to cook them.

Each stir-fry recipe is based upon the same principles and there are many different combinations you can try.

We stir-fry any vegetables that we can find sitting in the refrigerator. With larger vegetables such as cauliflower florets, the trick is to cut them fine enough so that they can cook within a three minute period. Here are a few suggestions, but don't be afraid to create your own combinations.

Mange-tout and Almond Stir-Fry (protein)

A delightful protein dish, thanks to the combination of delicate green mange-tout and crunchy almonds.

250 g (8 oz) mange-tout
30 ml (2 tbsp) soya oil
50 g (2 oz) almonds
(preferably blanched)

125 g (4 oz) button
mushrooms
5 ml (1 tsp) vegetable bouillon
powder

Top and tail the mange-tout. Heat oil in a wok or large frying pan and when hot add the almonds and stir-fry for three to five minutes. Then add the remaining ingredients and continue to stir-fry for another two to three minutes. Serve immediately.

Ultra-High Stir-Fry (neutral)

This neutral recipe is based on the sprouts – whatever sprouts you have will do nicely. Chinese mung-bean sprouts are traditionally used.

10 ml (2 tsp) soya oil
250 g (8 oz) mung sprouts or
other sprouted seeds or
grains

black pepper, freshly ground
1 large red pepper, deseeded
5 ml (1 tsp) vegetable bouillon
powder or soy sauce

Heat the oil in a wok or large frying pan. When hot, stir-fry the sprouts and pepper for one to two minutes. Add a little vegetable bouillon powder or soy sauce, season with black pepper, and serve immediately.

Green Stir-Fry (protein)

A lovely protein dish which goes well with a watercress salad.

15 ml (1 tbsp) soya oil
50 g (2 oz) cashew nuts or
   cashew-nut pieces
2 cloves garlic, chopped finely
250 g (8 oz) Chinese leaves,
   shredded
250 g (8 oz) broccoli florets

250 g (8 oz) green beans,
   sliced diagonally
5 ml (1 tsp) vegetable bouillon
   powder
15 ml (1 tbsp) spring or
   filtered water
juice of 1 lemon

Heat the oil in a wok or large frying pan. When hot, stir-fry the cashews and garlic for two to three minutes. Then add the vegetables and stir-fry for a further three to four minutes. Mix the vegetable bouillon powder with the water and lemon juice and pour over the vegetables and nuts and stir in well. Serve immediately.

Sesame-Courgette Stir-Fry (protein)

A light protein recipe which my son Jesse adores.

10 ml (2 tsp) sesame seed oil
   or soya oil
125 g (4 oz) sesame seeds
250 g (8 oz) courgettes

8 sticks of celery
250 g (8 oz) carrots
5 ml (1 tsp) vegetable bouillon
   powder or tamari

Cut up the vegetables into matchsticks. Heat the oil in a wok or large frying pan. When hot, add the sesame seeds and cook at a high heat for one to two minutes until they begin to brown. Then add the vegetables and cook for another two to three minutes. Season with bouillon powder or tamari and serve immediately.

Russian Red Stir-Fry (neutral)

A very light refreshing cabbage dish which is quick and easy to prepare.

350 g (¾ lb) red cabbage or
   Savoy cabbage
250 g (½ lb) white turnip
15 ml (1 tbsp) olive oil
4 spring onions, chopped
   finely
15 ml (1 tbsp) soy sauce

15 ml (1 tbsp) tomato purée
5 ml (1 tsp) cumin seeds
5 ml (1 tsp) paprika
5 ml (1 tsp) vegetable bouillon
   powder
freshly ground black pepper

Wash the cabbage and shred finely. Grate the turnip finely. Heat the oil in a large saucepan or wok and fry the cabbage–turnip mixture together with the spring onions over a high heat for three minutes. Add the remaining ingredients (including a little spring or filtered water if necessary) and cook for a further five minutes. Season with black pepper and serve immediately.

OTHER FAVOURITE VEGETABLE RECIPES

Artichokes (neutral)

Artichokes are one of my favourite vegetables. I like them served in almost any form. A simple vinaigrette sauce is perhaps best of all.

4 large artichokes
juice of ½ a lemon
sea-salt to taste

vinaigrette sauce or dip or
seed milk

Place the artichokes in a large pot of boiling water – at least 3 inch depth of water. Add the lemon juice and a pinch or two of sea-salt to season, and bring to the boil. Simmer for 45 minutes until the meat at the bottom of each artichoke leaf is softened. Remove and serve either hot or cold with a simple vinaigrette sauce or one of the richer dips or seed milks.

Corn on the Cob (starch)

4 corn-cobs
sea-salt to season

Tahini Mayonnaise dressing
(see page 116) or a little
butter and salt

Remove the corn husks and silk. Place the cobs in boiling, salted water and cook for 10–12 minutes. Strain and serve with Tahini Mayonnaise dressing or a little butter and salt.

Minty Peas (starch)

450 g (1 lb) fresh shelled
   garden peas
2.5 ml (½ tsp) vegetable
   bouillon powder
15 ml (1 tbsp) spring or

filtered water
30 ml (2 tbsp) fresh mint
(apple mint is particularly
good)

Put the peas into a pot with the water and vegetable bouillon powder and gently steam over a low heat for 15–20 minutes. Sprinkle with the mint for the last five minutes of cooking and serve immediately.

Pumpkin in Tahini (starch)

The small amount of tahini used here does not interfere with this starch vegetable and sets it off nicely.

1 large onion chopped finely
15 ml (1 tbsp) olive oil
15 ml (1 tbsp) tahini
450 g (1 lb) fresh pumpkin

(skin removed), cut into 1
inch cubes
2.5 ml (½ tsp) grated nutmeg

Sauté the onion in the oil until brown, then add the pumpkin and continue to sauté for 5–10 minutes, stirring carefully. Add a splash of water if necessary and leave on a very low heat for another 10–15 minutes until soft. Add the tahini and mix well. Serve immediately sprinkled with the grated nutmeg.

Easy Vegetable Curry (starch)

This takes no more than 20–30 minutes to prepare. It can be eaten on its own or with a light salad for supper. In smaller quantities serve as a side-dish for a living salad.

1 large onion, chopped finely
15 ml (1 tbsp) soya oil or
   olive oil or sunflower oil
10 ml (2 tsp) mild curry
   powder
3 large carrots, sliced
   tlengthways, then cut across
   to make 1½ inch sticks

1 medium-sized turnip, cut up
   finely into matchsticks
2 potatoes
5–7.5 ml (1-1½ tsp) vegetable
   bouillon powder
1½ C spring or filtered water
grated coconut (optional)

Sauté the onion in the oil until it becomes translucent, then add the curry powder and vegetable bouillon powder and continue to stir for a few minutes. Add the rest of the vegetables and pour in the water. Bring to the boil and simmer slowly for 20–30 minutes, then serve. It is particularly nice served with some grated dried coconut.

During the summer it's delightful to be able to add some French beans or some peas (I often like to add some chopped celery) – or, really, whatever other vegetables you have in the refrigerator.

Spicy Shish Kebab (neutral)

A delicious marinated, skewered vegetable dish which you can grill or barbecue. Serve it on a bed of brown rice cooked with vegetable bouillon powder and herbs. You will need two skewers for each person and it's a good idea to marinate the vegetables for two to four hours.

1 large aubergine, cut into 1¼ inch chunks
10 fresh tomatoes, halved
24 large mushrooms
1 red pepper
1 green pepper
2 large onions (preferably red), cut into 1 inch chunks
1 large swede or 2 small turnips, cut into 1 inch chunks

For the Marinade
1¼ C olive oil
juice from 3 lemons
30 ml (2 tbsp) red wine
3 cloves of garlic, crushed
5 ml (1 tsp) coriander, crushed
30 ml (2 tbsp) of parsley, finely chopped
2.5 ml (½ tsp) nutmeg, finely ground
15 ml (1 tbsp) fresh basil (optional)
2.5 ml (1 tsp) dried oregano

Wash, cut and prepare the vegetables. Place all the marinade ingredients together in a large bowl and mix thoroughly. Grill the aubergine until just soft and add with the rest of the vegetables to the marinade. Let it all sit for two to four hours. Skewer the vegetables, alternating from one to another, and baste them with the marinade as they are grilled or barbecued. May be served with a spicy sauce such as a tahini sauce, mayonnaise or chili sauce.

Aubergine Paté (protein)

I learned this recipe from a Middle Eastern friend who served it to me once. I had absolutely no idea what I was eating but found it completely irresistible. I have never forgotten the experience. You can vary the taste of it considerably by adding different spices or different extra ingredients.

2 medium aubergines
4 cloves of garlic, finely
  chopped
60 ml (4 tbsp) fresh parsley,
  finely chopped
1 small onion, finely chopped
½ C tahini

5 ml (1 tsp) vegetable bouillon
  powder or other seasoning
2.5 ml (½ tsp) ground cumin
pinch of cayenne
15 ml (1 tbsp) olive oil or
  Tahini Mayonnaise (see
  page 116)

Remove the stems from the aubergines and prick them with a fork as you would a potato. Put them into an oven and bake slowly until they become soft inside. Remove them, then scoop out the insides and put into a food processor to purée. Combine all the other ingredients (except the oil) in the food processor with the purée, remove and chill in a refrigerator. Pour the olive oil on top just before serving. You can use Tahini Mayonnaise instead of the olive oil as a delicious variation.

Vegi-stroganoff (protein)

A splendid protein-based vegetable dish that can be a real success for entertaining.

900–1150 g (2–2½ lb)
  chopped fresh vegetables
  (carrots, celery, courgettes,
  aubergine, cabbage,
  Chinese leaves, small
  tomatoes, cauliflower,
  broccoli, peas, etc.)

For the Sauce
1½ C raw cashews or cashew
  pieces
1½ C filtered or spring water
  (more if needed)

250 g (8 oz) chopped
  mushrooms
1 large onion, chopped finely
15 ml (1 tbsp) soya oil or
  olive oil
juice of 2 lemons
15 ml (3 tsp) vegetable
  bouillon powder
black pepper
1 ml (¼ tsp) dill
2.5–5 ml (½–1 tsp) paprika
45 ml (3 tbsp) dry red wine

To make the sauce, mince the cashew nuts finely in a food processor, then add the water and mix further into a creamy consistency. Sauté the mushrooms and onion in the oil until the onion is translucent. Then mix in all remaining sauce ingredients except the red wine. Cook very slowly, either in a double boiler or on a very slow burner. Then steam all the chopped vegetables in a little water. As soon as the vegetables are steamed, which usually takes 20–30 minutes, pour the sauce and wine over them, sprinkle with a dash of paprika and serve immediately.

Ginger Beans (starch)

5 ml (1 tsp) soya or other oil
450 g (1 lb) French beans
2 cloves garlic, chopped finely
15 ml (1 tbsp) fresh ginger, chopped finely

juice of 1 lemon
15 ml (1 tbsp) tamari or soy sauce

Put oil into a wok or large frying pan and heat. When hot, add vegetables, garlic and ginger and stir constantly. Cook for three to four minutes, season with tamari or soy sauce, and serve immediately.

Ratatouille (neutral)

A low-fat recipe which makes a delicious main meal eaten with either a protein or a starch salad. It's very filling.

2 large aubergines
1 large onion
4 cloves of garlic
15 ml (1 tbsp) olive oil
15 ml (1 tbsp) fresh basil or 5 ml (1 tsp) dried basil
450 g (1 lb) fresh skinned tomatoes or 450 g (15 oz) tin of tomatoes

1 large green pepper, deseeded and chopped
175 g (6 oz) fresh mushrooms
250 g (½ lb) courgettes, sliced
15 ml (1 tbsp) vegetable bouillon powder
freshly ground black pepper
45 ml (3 tbsp) chopped fresh parsley

Cut the aubergine into ½ inch cubes; chop the onion and the garlic finely. Heat the oil, then brown the aubergine, onion and garlic in the oil for five to ten minutes. Add the basil and cook for one more minute, then add tomatoes, green pepper, mushrooms, courgettes and bouillon powder and simmer for 25 minutes. Season with pepper and sprinkle with parsley. May be served either hot or chilled.

Braised Vegetables (starch)

This simple and inexpensive dish is a favourite with my son Aaron. It combines well with a living salad using a neutral or a starch dressing.

1 head of celery	5 ml (1 tsp) vegetable bouillon
6 medium potatoes	powder
5 large carrots	15 ml (1 tbsp) tahini
2 C spring or filtered water	freshly ground black pepper
1 bay leaf	

Scrub the vegetables and cut into strips about 3 inches long. Place in a large pot with water, bay leaf and vegetable bouillon powder; put into an oven pre-heated to 400°F (200°C), gas mark 6 and bake for 20 minutes. Add tahini and stir well, then replace in oven for a further five minutes. Season with black pepper and serve at once.

Baked Vegetables

I am extremely fond of baked vegetables because the process of baking seems to help the vegetables maintain their natural flavour. Besides, there is something quite charming to me about serving a whole baked onion at a meal: it's amusing as well as delicious.

Baking vegetables is one of the best methods of preserving their vitamins and minerals. You can bake vegetables either on their own or hidden within wholegrain pastry, or you can mix them together in a kind of hot-pot.

Jacket Potatoes (starch)

Baked potatoes make the most wonderful 'pockets' for salads, stir-fried vegetables, steamed vegetables and so forth. What you need to avoid are the traditional cheese, sour-cream, yogurt, etc., baked potato fillings because the combination of the starchy potato and the protein of cheese or

138

other dairy products is not a good one. However, there are many neutral vegetables and salads and dips that you can put into baked potatoes, from mashed avocados mixed together with some garlic and a little vegetable bouillon powder to a simple living salad of sprouts with a herbal dressing. One of my most favourite dishes of all is of baked potatoes which have been stuffed with such delicacies.

Pre-heat the oven to 400°F (200°C), gas mark 6. Scrub the potatoes carefully with a natural bristled brush but do not peel. Pierce the skins two or three times with a fork and bake for 1–1½ hours or until soft. Slit the potatoes open and fill with your desired filling – perhaps a little neutral salad dressing or a little mashed avocado and lemon. Baked potatoes are particularly delicious when sprinkled with fresh parsley which has been chopped finely.

Baked Leeks and Pecans (protein)

450 g (1 lb) leeks
15 ml (1 tbsp) soya oil or
other cooking oil
125 g (4 oz) pecans

30 ml (2 tbsp) miso
splash of spring or filtered
water

Slice the leeks lengthways in very fine strips and then cut into 3 inch lengths. Mix well with the oil and bake in a hot oven for 10–15 minutes. Chop the pecans finely in a food processor and combine with the miso and a little water to prepare a sauce for the leeks. Cover the leeks with the sauce and serve immediately.

Baked Carrots (protein)

6 large healthy carrots
30 ml (1 tbsp) olive oil or
soya oil

¼ C sesame seeds

Scrub the carrots well and slice them lengthways four or five times, then crossways into pieces about 3 inches long. Mix well with the oil, then place on a baking sheet and bake in a hot oven for 20 minutes. During the last 10 minutes of baking spread the sesame seeds over the top. Serve immediately.

Baked Parsnips (neutral)

450 g (1 lb) fresh parsnips
15–30 ml (1–2 tbsp) sesame
  oil or olive oil

2.5 ml (¹/2 tsp) vegetable
  bouillon powder
30 ml (2 tbsp) Dijon mustard

Slice the parsnips lengthways two or three times, then crossways into lengths about 3 inches long. Mix together the oil, the vegetable bouillon powder and the mustard and pour over to cover the parsnips. Bake in a moderate oven until golden brown – about 30–35 minutes.

Baked Turnips (neutral)

450 g (1 lb) fresh turnips
15–30 ml (1–2 tbsp) oil
5 ml (1 tsp) fresh ginger
2.5 ml (¹/2 tsp) vegetable
  bouillon powder

45 ml (3 tbsp) spring or
  filtered water

Cut the turnips into matchstick-sized strips and put into a casserole with the oil, the finely sliced ginger, the vegetable bouillon powder and the water. Cover with a lid and bake in a moderate oven until tender.

Baked Onions (neutral)

4 large Spanish onions

chopped parsley (as garnish)

Top and tail the onions but leave the outer skin on. Bake in a medium oven for 20–30 minutes until they are yielding to the touch. Take from the oven, remove the outer skins and serve immediately with a sprinkling of chopped parsley to garnish.

Chapter Nineteen

Gorgeous Grains

Six thousand years ago Zarathustra (Zoroaster), the Persian sage, waxed ecstatic about grains: 'When the light of the moon waxeth warmer,' he said, 'golden-hued grains grow up from the earth during the spring.' I think these words beautifully capture the richness and delight of the grain foods. Grains should always be eaten as close as possible to their natural state. The best way of all to eat them is sprouted. The next best is by cooking them slowly and eating them in side-dishes to go with living salads or supersalads.

The grains are rich in B-complex vitamins. And, providing they are unrefined, they are also rich in fibre. They are excellent foods for providing simple, long-sustained energy – as such, grain dishes play an important part in the diet of athletes. The leaner you become the more you will wish to increase the amount of grains you are eating.

Here are a few simple grain recipes to get you started.

Yummy Brown Rice (starch)
Rice cooked in this manner is so delicious that it seems to be a worthwhile dish in itself. It needs no special sauces or condiments to make it work.

1 C brown rice
2–3 C spring or filtered water
15 ml (1 tbsp) olive oil
10 ml (2 tsp) vegetable
   bouillon powder

15 ml (3 tbsp) fresh parsley,
   chopped
5 ml (1 tsp) pot marjoram
2 cloves garlic, finely chopped
   (optional)

Wash the rice three times under running water and put into a saucepan. Boil the water in a kettle and pour over the rice. Add seasonings except for 1 tbsp of the parsley. Bring to the boil and cook gently for 45 minutes or until all the liquid has been absorbed. Garnish with parsley and serve. (You can double this recipe and prepare enough rice to make a large rice salad the next day.)

Kasha (starch)

A favourite of the Russians, kasha is also a favourite of mine. It is quick to cook and has a pleasant nutty flavour.

2 C buckwheat groats
spring or filtered water to
   cover
10 ml (2 tsp) vegetable
   bouillon powder

30 ml (2 tbsp) chopped fresh
   parsley or other herbs

Place buckwheat in a heavy-bottomed pan and roast it dry over a medium heat while stirring with a wooden spoon. As it begins to darken pour hot water over the buckwheat and add the vegetable bouillon powder and 1 tbsp of the herbs. Cover and simmer very slowly for 15–20 minutes until all the liquid has been absorbed. Serve with the remaining herbs sprinkled on the top.

Polenta (starch)

Polenta is a peasant dish made from cornmeal. I particularly like it served with a living salad dressed with a spicy sauce which I put on the polenta as well.

3 C filtered or spring water
1 C cornmeal

10 ml (2 tsp) vegetable
   bouillon powder or tamari

Heat the water in a kettle. Pour boiling water over the cornmeal and blend into a paste with the vegetable bouillon powder or tamari. Stir until smooth and cook very gently until all the liquid has been absorbed. Cool and drop by the spoonful on to a slightly oiled baking sheet and grill until brown turning once.

Millet (starch)

Once used by the Romans to make porridge, millet is still an important staple in many parts of Africa. It is a bland and highly nutritious grain which contains all of the essential amino acids plus an excellent complement of the B-complex vitamins and minerals.

5 C spring or *filtered water*
1 C millet
10 ml (2 tsp) vegetable
  bouillon powder
1 medium onion, chopped
  finely

5 ml (1 tsp) paprika
30 ml (2 tbsp) chopped
  parsley, fresh

Boil the water and pour it over the millet in a deep saucepan; then add the vegetable bouillon powder, onion, paprika and half of the parsley. Cook over slow heat for 30–45 minutes until all of the liquid has been absorbed. Sprinkle with the remainder of the parsley and serve. (Cooked millet can be formed into small balls together with grated carrots, finely chopped onions, a little parsley and a little lemon juice and served cold as part of a salad.)

Barley Pilaff (starch)

A delicious baked dish which goes nicely with a living salad. It is made from pot barley, not from pearl barley (too many of the B-complex vitamins and minerals have been removed from pearl barley). Barley is also excellent used in soups.

2 onions, chopped finely
15 ml (1 tbsp) soya or *olive oil*
1 C pot barley
1½ C spring or *filtered water*
15 ml (1 tbsp) vegetable
  bouillon powder

15 ml (1 tbsp) dill
2 cloves of garlic, finely
  chopped (optional)

Sauté the onions in the oil until translucent, then add the barley, continuing to stir until the grains have become well coated. Remove from the heat and add the remaining ingredients (including the water, boiled in a kettle). Place in a well-oiled oven dish and bake in a moderate oven for half an hour. Check to see if you need to add a little more water. Serve immediately.

Perfect Oatmeal Porridge (starch)

A superb starch meal and an absolute delight to eat in the evening because the high carbohydrate content of porridge has a tendency to increase the brain's uptake of the amino acid tryptophan and therefore to relax you.

1 C porridge oats　　　　　　*1 ripe banana*
3 C spring or *filtered water*　*5 ml (1 tsp) cinnamon*
pinch of sea salt

Preferably soak the oats for several hours before cooking (you can put them in the pot with the water at lunchtime if the porridge is to be prepared for your evening meal). Heat the porridge and water in a double boiler or place the pan containing the oats and water itself into a large frying pan which contains 2 inches of water. This means that the porridge will cook very slowly and be very smooth. Cook slowly for 15–20 minutes until the mixture has become smooth. If you prefer a thicker mixture you can reduce the amount of water. Remove from stove and pour into a dish with sliced bananas and sprinkle with cinnamon. Serve immediately.

Chapter Twenty

On the Go

So there you have it – the principles, the rationale, the guidelines, the recipes and all the rest. Now it is only a question of putting it all into practice and sitting back to enjoy the transformations that are going to take place in your body. But what about special circumstances? For instance, how do you make Raw Energy Food Combining work for you when you have to eat in restaurants, or when you are travelling, or if you want to take your lunch to work or to school with you? It is all a lot easier to cope with than you might imagine.

Lunch is East

The business lunch or evening out needn't be a problem. These days more and more restaurants serve decent salads. And, while it is true that most of them are not exactly living delights, they are still a far cry from the traditional limp piece of lettuce with a slice of cucumber, half a tomato and a pale hard-boiled egg.

If you want to eat fish or meat or game then order a dish which is *simply* prepared – not smothered in breadcrumbs (bad starch–protein combination) – such as trout or prawns. If it comes with rice or potatoes ask the waiter if you could please have some vegetables instead and then a mixed or green salad. You can also always order fruit juice or fruit as a starter, provided you leave 20 minutes or more before you start on your next course.

If, like me, you prefer most of the time to stick to vegetable foods, you might order a light green salad to start with and follow that with a plate of whatever the vegetables of the day are. The better the restaurant the more helpful they will be. Most of the time you will be able to order without anybody even suspecting that you are practising conscientious food combining.

If, again like me, you prefer to remain as inconspicuous in your dieting as possible, then it is a good idea to order the same number of courses as the other people you are dining with. You could choose an avocado vinaigrette to start with, for instance, followed by a game main course, some vegetables, and a side salad. Nobody will oblige you to eat pudding these days. I sometimes carry some peppermint tea bags with me as an after-dinner drink while friends are drinking coffee. Then I simply order 'a small pot of tea without the tea please' and pop my bag into it to steep for a couple of minutes when it arrives. By all means enjoy a glass of good wine if you want one.

Friends Can Help

When I was a child my father always accused me of 'stirring my food around my plate' instead of eating it. He is the only person I have ever known who actually noticed that I do this. And it is a great technique to practise when you are in a situation where food combinations have been put on your plate which you do not want to eat (this frequently happens to me at dinner parties). The best way to deal with it is to decide whether you are going to make your meal a protein one or a starch one and then eat only the foods in your selected category, simply moving the rest about on your plate so they look well picked over. When your hostess offers you seconds you can reply with, 'Yes, I would love some more of that delicious rice', or 'Do you think I could have another serving of salad; it's wonderful?' At dinner parties make sure you eat plenty of the side-salads, the vegetables and whatever other neutral foods are available. And don't be afraid to say 'no thank you' when people become persistent with their offers. You can always add, 'It looks lovely but I'm afraid I'm rather full.'

Fly Away

This is easiest of all. Travelling on planes, in the car or on trains is the ideal time to spend a day on fruit or to apple-fast. Not only is it convenient, because you have a ready-made opportunity for not following the standard pattern of three meals a day, it will also help your stamina and your ability to withstand the stress of getting from here to there very well indeed. I never get on an aeroplane for a long flight without a bag of fruit under my arm. Usually it is the most luscious fruit I can find, since I tend rather to spoil myself on the excuse that 'after all, I'm travelling today and so it's rather a special time'. Most airlines these days offer special meals which fit in well with your needs – for instance, fresh fruit salads with yogurt or cottage cheese, or seafood salads: you need only request them 24 hours before your flight. Once you get used to growing your own sprouts you may even want to carry some of those with you on the go. We often do – especially when we are out hiking (they will grow in plastic bags in a rucksack as well as they do in jars in your kitchen) or when there is a long car journey.

Take It Out

Raw vegetables, fruits or sprouts make excellent foods to put in a lunchbox for school or work. For instance, you can combine any crudités – carrot sticks, celery sticks, broccoli and cauliflower florets, rings or strips of red, yellow and green peppers, mange-tout, diagonal slices of cucumber, courgette, thin slices of Jerusalem artichoke, white radish, kohlrabi, button mushrooms, spring onions, celery hearts, tomatoes, watercress – with a container of rich protein dressing or dip. This makes a delightful lunch. And, provided you keep your fresh vegetables on hand in the refrigerator all cleaned and ready for use as I do, the whole thing will take you no more than five to ten minutes to prepare.

For most people following a Raw Energy Food Combining lifestyle from day to day, being out and about presents little problem. You will probably find after the first few weeks, once you have got the hang of food combining and know pretty well what goes with what, you will not even have to think much about it. After all, if ever things go wrong and you find yourself having eaten a badly combined meal, you can always make the next day an all-raw one or an apple-fast to get yourself back in balance again.

New Life Starts Here

The extraordinary thing about Raw Energy Food Combining is that, once you do get into it, once you have shed your unwanted fat, enhanced your energy levels and are feeling in top form, chances are you are going to want to stick with it. When your body has re-adjusted itself to its normal weight you can begin to experiment a little. Keep to your food combining but now try eating a few more of your foods cooked. Add more grains to your meals. Try the pulses again, for by now your digestive system will probably have become so much more efficient and so much stronger that you will be able to handle them without difficulty. You will see for yourself how easy it is to take everything you have learned as well as all the positive changes which have happened to you through new ways of eating and exercising and slowly build for yourself a lasting lifestyle for health and good looks. That, after all, is what Raw Energy Food Combinining is all about.

Resources

Food Processor: Magimix processors are the best available.

Herb Teas: Some of my favourite blends include Cinnamon Rose, Orange Zinger, and Emperor's Choice by Celestial Seasonings; Warm & Spicy by Symmingtons; and Creamy Carob French Vanilla. Yogi Tea, by Golden Temple Products, is a strong spicy blend, perfect as a coffee replacement.

Honey: The Garvin Honey Company have a good selection of set and clear honeys from all over the world. These can be ordered from The Garvin Honey Company Ltd, Garvin House, 158 Twickenham Road, Isleworth, Middlesex, TW7 7LD. Tel: 0181 560 7171. The New Zealand Natural Food Company have a fine range of honey, including organic honey, in particular Manuka honey, known for its anti-bacterial effects. The New Zealand Natural Food Company Ltd, Holt Close, Highgate Wood, London, N10 3HW. Tel: 0181 444 5660

Juice Extractor: Moulinex do an inexpensive centrifugal juicer which is good.

Living Foods Workshops: Naturopath, Elaine Bruce, who has spent eighteen years working with living foods as a tool for healing, and teaching how to make delicious recipes, offers an intensive training in her own approach to health and vitality. The complete programme takes two weekends 9:30AM to 5PM each day and includes many raw food goodies as well as raw feast lunches. Or you can choose to do only the first weekend.

For further information contact Elaine Bruce, Living Foods and Natural Medicine, Holmleigh, 49 Gravel Hill, Ludlow SY8 1QS. Tel: 01584 875308.

Marigold Low Salt Swiss Vegetable Bouillon Powder: This instant broth powder based on vegetables and herbs is available from healthfood stores or direct from Marigold Foods, Unit 10, St Pancras Commercial Centre, 63 Pratt Street, London, NW1 0BY. Tel: 0171 267 7368.

Organic Meat: Good quality organic beef, pork, bacon, lamb, chicken, a variety of types of sausage, and a selection of cheeses, can be ordered from Eastbrook Farm Organic Meats, Bishopstone, Swindon, Wiltshire, SN6 8PW. Tel: 01793 790 460, fax: 01793 791 239. All goods are sent for next day delivery, vacuum packed and chilled.

Sea Plants: such as kelp, dulse, nori, kombu, can be bought from Japanese grocers or macrobiotic health shops.

Index